PROSTrATE
CANCER

Also by Graham Sharpe

A Gentleman's Guide to Calculating Winning Bets
– A Sporting Ready Reckoner

1001 Great Gambling Tips

Dorothy Paget – The Eccentric Queen of the Sport of Kings

(with Declan Colley)

William Hill – The Man & The Business

(with Mihir Bose)

The Man Who Was Screaming Lord Sutch

Free the Manchester United One – The Inside Story of
Football's Greatest Scam

The Magnificent Seven – How Frankie Dettori Achieved the Impossible

Vinyl Countdown

PROSTrATE CANCER

THE MISUNDERSTOOD MALE KILLER

Graham Sharpe

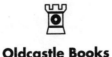

Oldcastle Books

First published in 2022 by Oldcastle Books
Harpenden, Herts, UK
www.oldcastlebooks.co.uk

A CIP catalogue record for this book is available from the British Library.

ISBN:
978-0-85730-462-9 (Paperback)
978-0-85730-463-6 (eBook)

2 4 6 8 10 9 7 5 3 1

Typeset in 11 on 13.4pt Goudy Old Style
by Avocet Typeset, Bideford, Devon, EX392BP
Printed and bound in Great Britain by CPI Group (UK) Ltd, Croydon, CR0 4YY

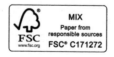

THIS BOOK IS DEDICATED
to anyone who believes there are two 'R's in PROSTATE –
I hope you don't have to learn the hard way how to tell
your 'R's from your elbow!

CONTENTS

Letter in the Metro, *25 June 2021*

'I have lost count of the number of friends I know who
have complained of "prostrate" problems. I have
stopped bothering to correct them.'
– Ben Mundy, of Wells, Somerset.

FOREWORD

WHEN GRAHAM told me he had been diagnosed with Prostate Cancer it was at first a shock, but after I had taken the news in, all the previous GP and hospital visits he had been taking made sense.

He did not want anyone to be told, which I really didn't like at all. That was something that I couldn't do. So I made the decision to tell our two sons.

Our elder son, Steeven, lives in New Zealand, and we were going there to see him and his family for Christmas and New Year. I told him shortly after we arrived, and he took the news very well.

I then told Paul when we returned home, and it was agreed that when I updated him on G's treatment and how he was feeling, he would keep Steeven in the loop.

This worked very well, and I felt much better, knowing that they were aware of what was happening. Graham was completely unaware that I had told them, but I felt then, and still feel now, that what I did was the right thing to do.

And now he knows what I did – as I have just told him.

Sheila Sharpe

INTRODUCTION

IN WHICH I PROSTRATE MYSELF

I VAGUELY recall having read an article many years ago, one phrase of which stuck in my memory: 'Most people affected by the disease will die *with* prostate cancer, rather than *from* it.' Thus it had never occurred to me to worry about the consequences of being diagnosed with prostate cancer, or 'PC', as I have come to call it. As a result of having read that article I did, though, at least become aware of the spelling and pronunciation of the word 'prostate'.

Very few people – none, as far as I can recall – have ever told me of the time they found themselves or someone else prostate on the ground. Those who wish to, almost invariably use the correct word for that phrase – 'prostrate'. There seems to be little confusion about the correct usage of the word prostrate in these circumstances. But many people have spoken to me about themselves or others being a victim of 'prostrate cancer'.

I wonder why it is that a comparatively significant percentage of those who find themselves having to deal with the condition, or who are speaking of others who already have it, appear to struggle to name it correctly. I don't find it disrespectful or upsetting when people use the wrong terminology, but it does strike me that perhaps there is an unwillingness amongst men of a certain age, predominantly those who are not suffering from this extremely common cancer amongst males of advancing years, to confront it. To the extent that they either genuinely do not, cannot, or will not absorb the pronunciation of the disease they fear that they, too, may find themselves having to deal with at some stage of their lives.

When those who are diagnosed with PC endure the ritual of

confirmation, they may be temporarily shocked into a state of mind which doesn't want to take in the enormity of what they are being told. Or they may feel that they have no intention of recognising the severity of the position into which they have just been inserted, for fear of the next step being to accept the potentially fatal consequences. Perhaps part of their rejection of the concept of having the disease manifests as not allowing its name to register. Or maybe – and this seems very unlikely – there are just too many hard of hearing, and/or illiterate men who are diagnosed with what they hear as prostrate cancer, possibly by less than clearly enunciating doctors, medics, specialists, consultants or oncologists.

Whether one calls it prostate or prostrate won't affect the ultimate outcome, but, get it right, and at least you won't be accused of not even knowing what you've been diagnosed with. Unless the accusation comes from someone who believes it really is called prostrate cancer, of course...

1

IN WHICH MS MCNULTY BECOMES MY HEROINE

'COME IN, Mr Sharpe... sit down... I have to tell you that you have prostate cancer... Oh, would you excuse me? I'm on call today...'

The consultant stood up to answer his ringing mobile, and walked out of the room, while I sat trying to process what he'd just told me. He returned shortly after and began to tell me about his diagnosis: 'Sorry about that, Mr Sharpe. Where was I? Ah yes, you have prostate cancer, and...'

His mobile was ringing again. 'Sorry, I have to take this, I'm on call...' He stood up again, and, speaking into the mobile, left the room.

I'm not usually backward about coming forward, and when this happened yet again, I was thinking, 'I'm really not happy about this. He may be on call, but for all I know he's just told me I have a death sentence hanging over me, and he can't be bothered to turn his phone off. I won't be responsible for my actions if he does it again.'

The Macmillan nurse who had also been sitting quietly in the room with us must have sensed my possibly murderous thoughts.

'Okay, come with me, Mr Sharpe, I'll explain what he should be telling you.' She walked out of the room, and I followed her into her office across the corridor. I never saw the consultant again...

In all probability, this will not be the way in which, if it is going to happen to you – and the chances are relatively high that it could, if you are male and aged 50-plus – the news will be broken. Much more likely is that you will find out as Ron Arnold did, someone I hadn't known prior to the pair of us eventually sitting close to each other in a waiting room in Mount Vernon Cancer Centre, waiting to undergo our radiotherapy treatment. We would soon become firm friends.

It was Thursday 4 October 2018, that Ron, then 73 years old, went to his 4pm appointment to be told the results from the biopsy he had recently undergone: 'We sat down in his consulting room. He had a serious face. Can't remember his exact words. Something like: "Mr Arnold, I'm afraid it has been confirmed that you have prostate cancer".'

Ron remembers that he responded to the news with something like, 'Okay, I thought so – what do we do next?'

He was told 'that the next procedure should be a bone scan to make sure that it has not spread – if it has it will require a totally different type of treatment.' Ron replied: 'Okay, now it has been established that I have it... How will I react, and how is it going to be dealt with?'

Stay with me and you'll find out how Ron and I got on...

Just a day or two after my bluntly, brutally and insensitively delivered consultant's verdict, I received a letter dated 16 August 2018 from Fiona McNulty (*sic*), my Macmillan urology nurse and a copy of what she had written to my GP, Dr K, informing him of my 'Cancer Diagnosis: Prostate-C61.'

As I write this two and a half years later, I still have no idea what C61 means, so I google it, and up comes the following information: '**C61** is a "billable" ICD code used to specify a diagnosis of malignant neoplasm of prostate. A "billable code" is detailed enough to be used to specify a medical diagnosis.'

That's interesting, but leaves me very little the wiser, so I google 'malignant neoplasm of prostate'... then wish I hadn't, when I read this: 'A malignant neoplasm is basically cancer. Of the various types of neoplasm, this is the most severe as it can invade surrounding organs and tissues and also spread to other parts of the body through metastasis. During this process, cells break off of the neoplasm and travel through the blood vessels to other parts of the body.' Sounds a little daunting. I'm glad I didn't know that when I started my treatment...

Next, my googling informs me that: 'The five stages of prostate cancer are Sky, Teal, Azure, Indigo, and Royal.' A little more research shows that the fact that the initials of these stages spell out STAIR is not coincidental. They also gradually rise in potential severity.

Then up comes: 'Here are five potential warning signs of prostate cancer: A painful or burning sensation during urination or ejaculation. Frequent urination, particularly at night. Difficulty stopping or starting urination. Sudden erectile dysfunction. Blood in urine or semen.' Yes, I had had a couple of those.

The very thorough Ms McNulty, whose actions had avoided an unpleasant scene with the uncaring consultant, had made careful notes and sent me a copy of the 'Concerns' she had raised with me after removing me from the danger zone:

Level of distress the patient has been feeling (0 = low, 10 = extreme): **1**
Work concerns: **No concerns**
Grocery shopping (I might possibly have given her a slightly misleading impression here as she wrote...): **No concerns, does all own shopping and cooking** (Please, please, don't tell Sheila will you...?!)
Bathing or dressing: **No concerns**
Relationship with partner: **No concerns, lives with supportive wife** (Phew, I gave the right answer there, anyway...)
Passing urine: **No concerns**
Eating or appetite: **No concerns**
Hot flushes: **No complaints of hot flushes since starting the hormones. No concerns**
Moving around: **Fully mobile. No concerns**
Other medical condition: **On waiting list to have a gallbladder operation, no concerns**
Fatigue: **No complaints since starting the hormones. No concerns**

All those 'no concerns' made me think, well, yes, I do actually have a few concerns, but probably best to keep them to myself.

2

IN WHICH I WONDER HOW I HAD REACHED THIS POINT

MY EARLIEST indication of literally internal rumblings arrived on 11 December 2017, when I received a briefing on the results of an abdominal ultrasound which, wrote my GP, 'show uncomplicated gallstones. In the light of these results we would suggest having a discussion about a surgical referral – and avoiding fatty foods as far as possible in the interim.' Apparently, I was later informed, 'uncomplicated' didn't necessarily mean uncomplicated. I may have got the wrong end of the stick, of course.

The best part of a year later, in October 2018, my gallbladder had left the building. More accurately, had been left in the building – the Central Middlesex Hospital. However, this satisfactory outcome did not mean that I could resume a life untroubled by medical issues, as I was now being gradually drawn into the process of receiving treatment for prostate cancer, although the medics had been happy that this shouldn't delay the gallbladder removal as there was no direct correlation.

This newer situation had begun to reveal itself in early May 2018 when I learned that a urine sample I'd submitted did 'show blood'. There was more on this subject from my trusted GP, who wrote: 'The prostate does need to be checked via a blood test, then an appointment to see me.'

I duly took the PSA test and on 15 May 2018 was told: 'Unfortunately the PSA has come back elevated (it was, I discovered, 40.46, which is not recommended) and this needs urgent further evaluation. I have taken the liberty of making an urgent referral to urology to investigate this further.' Says the NHS: 'The PSA test is a blood test to help detect Prostate Cancer. But it's not perfect and will not help find all Prostate Cancers'.

It obviously was pretty urgent as I had an outpatient appointment scheduled at the Central Middlesex Hospital on 22 May – although, if I'm honest, I can't now recall whether this was gallbladder or prostate-related, or a combination of both. But the next appointment was on 12 June at Northwick Park Hospital for a 'Urology Flexible Cystoscopy'.

Mmm. That was something else.

Interestingly, the 'consent form' I had to sign began with a 'Name of Procedure' section which insisted they should 'include brief explanation if medical term not clear'.

I got no explanation, but while I was disrobing prior to it being my turn, the chap before me, rather younger than my 67, walked into the changing room. He couldn't stop laughing, in a slightly hysterical manner. 'Oh, man,' he said, looking at me and laughing some more, 'Oh, man.'

A few minutes later, I knew exactly what he meant and was also feeling that the best way to cope with the situation was, indeed, slightly hysterical, disbelieving laughter, but minus the usual warm feeling which accompanies genuine guffawing.

You want to know what happened, don't you? The official description is: 'a telescopic examination of the lining of the bladder via the urethra (urinary tube). A local anaesthetic jelly is used to numb and lubricate the urethra to make passage into the bladder as comfortable (me, on reading this later – 'hah!!') as possible. Most patients experience some discomfort during the procedure (me – if you are one of those who apparently doesn't/didn't, kindly write to me, care of the publisher. I have zero anticipation that anyone will fit this description of experiencing no discomfort.) but the majority do not find it too troublesome.'

No, I didn't find it too 'troublesome', but sitting there, aware of what was actually happening, really did cause one to think, '*Is this actually happening?'* Even now, a couple of years down the line, writing this I'm thinking: 'Seriously? They really did that? And I sat calmly and permitted them to do it!'

They also explained to me that I had to drink plenty of fluids for the next two days, and that for the next three or four I might find when passing urine that it would sting or burn slightly, and that my urine might be 'slightly bloodstained', but that all of this would 'clear rapidly'.

And you know what? It did. It was. It cleared.

If that experience didn't completely break my spirit, the one on 3 July 2018 for a 'US-guided biopsy prostate transrectal' came close to doing so – but for the intervention of a Kiwi nurse. The consent form offered a hand-written clue. Under the heading: 'Serious or frequently occurring risks' was scribbled: 'BLEEDING, INFECTION, PAIN.' And for suffering the risks thus described, what were 'the intended benefits'? 'DIAGNOSIS.'

Of course, I signed on the dotted line, then sat down amongst a small group of fellow victims to await the inevitable. I was the last to be seen.

If you don't particularly want to know the gory details of what happened, I would advise skipping the next couple of paragraphs, which explain the procedure:

'A small ultrasound probe is inserted into your back passage. The probe is slightly wider and longer than a finger. It is important to try and relax as this will make the test less uncomfortable. The doctor can then see an image of the prostate gland on a screen. You will be given a local anaesthetic injection into the prostate gland through the probe. Some small samples of tissue (biopsies) of the prostate gland are then taken, also through the probe. This can be uncomfortable but is not painful. The test should take about 20 minutes.'

Twenty minutes. That's about half of the playing time of an LP.
'The biopsies can be negative – no cancer seen. This is good

news...' But don't get too excited, though as: 'It is possible to miss very tiny areas of cancer in a set of biopsies.'

Then: 'The biopsies may be positive. Not so good news.'

After the procedure you're told to rest for a while. The info sheet suggested 15-20 minutes was appropriate, adding that it was 'probably inadvisable to drive immediately after the test. Please drink some extra glasses of water each day for a few days.'

We were all told we couldn't depart until we'd urinated after the test. Eventually I was the last patient left. I'd begun chatting with the New Zealand nurse. I have family in New Zealand. She had been exiled for some years, if I recall. I became aware that as soon as I was done she could go home, although not to New Zealand, of course. I began to feel guilty for keeping her waiting, even though she showed absolutely no signs of wanting me gone.

It took me a couple of hours to be able to go, before I could go... I'll always remember that nurse's patience and empathy. I know what a cliché it is to overpraise medics, and of course our emotions are heightened by our fears and state of mind at the time. But she was genuinely the difference between me heading home in a confused stupor and being able to do so in a calm, collected fashion, satisfied that one of my worst experiences was now, literally, behind me...

This is from the NHS website (in December 2020):

There's currently no screening programme for prostate cancer in the UK. This is because it has not been proved that the benefits would outweigh the risks.

PSA screening

Routinely screening all men to check their prostate-specific antigen (PSA) levels is a controversial subject in the international medical community. There are several reasons for this.

PSA tests are unreliable and can suggest prostate cancer when no cancer exists (a false-positive result). Most men are now offered an

MRI scan before a biopsy to help avoid unnecessary tests, but some men may have invasive, and sometimes painful, biopsies for no reason.

Furthermore, up to 15% of men with prostate cancer have normal PSA levels (a false-negative result), so many cases may be missed.

The PSA test can find aggressive prostate cancer that needs treatment, but it can also find slow-growing cancer that may never cause symptoms or shorten life. Some men may face difficult decisions about treatment, although this is less likely now that most men are offered an MRI scan before further tests and treatment.

Treating prostate cancer in its early stages can be beneficial in some cases, but the side effects of the various treatments are potentially so serious that men may choose to delay treatment until it's absolutely necessary.

Although screening has been shown to reduce a man's chance of dying from prostate cancer, it would mean many men receive treatment unnecessarily.

More research is needed to determine whether the possible benefits of a screening programme would outweigh the harms of:

- overdiagnosis – people being diagnosed with a cancer that would never cause symptoms or shorten life expectancy
- overtreatment – people being treated unnecessarily for tumours that would unlikely be harmful

What's a raised PSA level?
The amount of PSA in your blood is measured in nanograms of PSA per millilitre of blood (ng/ml).

If you're aged 50 to 69, raised PSA is 3ng/ml or higher.

A raised PSA level in your blood may be a sign of prostate cancer, but it can also be a sign of another condition that's not cancer, such as:

- an enlarged prostate
- prostatitis
- urinary infection

How accurate is the PSA test?
About 3 in 4 men with a raised PSA level will not have cancer. The PSA test can also miss about 15% of cancers.

Pros and cons of the PSA test

Pros:

- it may reassure you if the test result is normal
- it can find early signs of cancer, meaning you can get treated early
- PSA testing may reduce your risk of dying if you do have cancer

Cons:

- it can miss cancer and provide false reassurance
- it may lead to unnecessary worry and medical tests when there's no cancer
- it cannot tell the difference between slow-growing and fast-growing cancers
- it may make you worry by finding a slow-growing cancer that may never cause any problems

Friday 10 August had been on my mind while I was on holiday, and on that precise date I duly put in an appearance at Northwick Park's Isotope Scanning facility for my 'NM bone whole body' Isotope scan.

Radioactive liquid was injected into a vein in my arm – no, couldn't tell you which.

'You will be required to drink extra fluids and empty your bladder regularly between the injection and the pictures.'

Then I was called to see Dr A on Monday 24 September at 2.20pm at Northwick Park. This resulted in Dr A sending me a copy of the letter she sent to the consultant urological surgeon, Mr Giles Hellawell, telling him: 'We have been through the rationale, practicalities and expected side-effects of radical radiotherapy to the prostate and pelvis. He will need to remain on LHRH analogues for a minimum of two years. He is due to have the cholecystectomy (surgical removal of the gallbladder) in October and therefore we have agreed to meet in November to plan his radiotherapy for the New Year.' That was all accurate but like, I suspect, many other patients, when I'd had meetings with Dr A I'd heard and agreed with what she'd told me, but found it difficult afterwards to retain the information she'd given me, other than in the vaguest detail.

As Santa was preparing for his busiest evening of the year, I received good tidings from the Mount Vernon Cancer Centre, dated 24 December 2018, whose anonymous 'secretary to clinician' was writing to confirm that an outpatient appointment had been arranged for me to be seen at the Mount Vernon Cancer Centre 'under the care of: Dr A on 14 January 2019 at 14.30 in MVRG/ GEN1'.

Happy New Year to me, eh?

There followed copious information about how to access the relevant car park and a semi-upper case warning that 'PARKING FINES' were 'in operation'. This possible harbinger of doom was only slightly diluted by a reminder to bring the letter along with me 'to provide confirmation that' I was 'a patient receiving treatment in the Cancer Centre to receive a reduced rate parking token'. What a relief to learn that acquiring a Premier League medical complaint entitled me to pay less than other merely fit mortals to park my car.

Of course, I had a trump card to play here – my Freedom Pass, acquired via great age, entitling me to completely free travel on the buses and Tube trains which could put me adjacent to the Mount Vernon car parks and in a position to guffaw and snigger at the poor car-bound travellers forced to shell out to attend their cancer treatment.

Three hours before the meeting with Dr A, though, I was 'invited' to attend a Pre-radiotherapy Group Information consultation, which was to last about an hour and end with refreshments at the on-site Lynda Jackson Macmillan Cancer Centre, a drop-in Centre for patients to talk and ask questions about all aspects of cancer and its treatments. We were indeed given a chatty welcome, herded around and shown where we would be receiving our treatment, and invited to ask questions.

It was a good PR exercise, but how much actual knowledge any of us acquired would be open to discussion. Although I enjoyed the cup of tea afterwards, it would be the last time that I would enter the Lynda Jackson Centre – no, I wasn't banned, I just didn't really think it offered anything that I specifically needed at the time. I would, though, certainly not try to prevent anyone else from taking full advantage of the facilities. It would definitely not be sensible to dismiss it without checking it out first, either.

Whilst there we were handed a great deal of bumpf from Macmillan, offering all sorts of information about all aspects of PC – including something I never ever plucked up the courage to use... The Macmillan Toilet Card...

'You can use this card during or after treatment. If you need to use a toilet urgently, you can show it in places such as shops, offices, cafes and pubs.' ...yes, I'm sure one could, but equally, I just never would. This is purely a result of my own ridiculous self-esteem. I genuinely could not bring myself to admit in public that I was so likely to wet myself that I had to produce a card to prove it, thus doubly embarrassing myself!

Of course, I have kept the card 'just in case' I might ever need to use it and be so drunk I'd dare to... Please don't emulate this totally foolish attitude should you ever be offered a 'Toilet Card'. There's nothing to be ashamed about in requiring to use one. Bear in mind that in late November, 2021, it was revealed that one in five public toilets in the land have been closed over the past six years.

A couple of hours later I was seeing Dr A, who was very reassuring about the treatment I would be undergoing. I think she liked me, mind you. Well, I saw a couple of letters she'd written to my GP about me, in which she'd written, 'It was a pleasure to see Mr Sharpe...' and 'It was a pleasure to speak with Graham today...' As well as calling me 'this gentleman'.

Nor was she alone in this positively positive attitude towards me. A clinical oncology specialist who wrote about me declared: 'It was a pleasure to meet Mr Sharpe...' A locum consultant surgeon penned this: 'Thank you very much for allowing me to see this pleasant 69-year-old gentleman...' While yet another medic agreed: 'It was a pleasure to review Mr Sharpe...' Nor must I overlook the consultant orthopaedic surgeon I also visited: 'Many thanks for sending this nice man up.' His comment may have unknowingly told the truth – they were all just sending me up!

Clearly, though, all of these medical experts are instructed and/ or trained to write their letters in a specific manner, and to ensure they compliment and respect their patients along the way. I have to admit that it does encourage the patient to think well of them – except, of course, for the arrogant, unfeeling bas*ard who broke the news that I had PC to me so gently.

3

IN WHICH THE PROBLEM BECOMES APPARENT

THE GENESIS of this book was the operation to remove my gallbladder in October 2018. In the build-up to this, I had to undergo various tests and procedures, being poked, probed and prodded innumerable times, all the while not having much idea precisely what each succeeding investigation was being done for, but knowing it was likely to lead to a conclusion as to whether or not I would be retaining the gallbladder, to which I had become rather attached over the past 60-plus years.

I wondered whether not only the imminent gallbladder operation would need to be cancelled, but also our scheduled trip to New Zealand to see our two-year-old granddaughter. The unanimous decision by the medics I asked was that neither should be. That in itself made me feel a little better about the PC which they clearly didn't think was about to carry me off to my coffin.

My ignorance of medical matters was pretty much complete at this time. Not since the removal of a cartilage during the 1970s had I been admitted to hospital and my health had been consistently good overall. There had been a couple of small ops for carpal tunnel syndrome, one for each hand, but they didn't even involve overnight stays.

However, after experiencing stomach discomfort sufficient to prevent me being able to join friends and family dining out on several occasions, I had realised there was almost certainly something not quite right. I was right that things weren't right, which was how I ended up in the Central Middlesex Hospital, being de-gallbladdered.

This did involve an overnight stay in hospital, partially because when I was taken in to be operated on, an important-looking part of the equipment on which I was lying fell off unexpectedly. Blank looks all round in the theatre, but it was eventually repaired – or stuck back on – and I was duly anaesthetised and deprived of the gallbladder, albeit by then too late to be sent home that night.

Five days later I was in Liverpool with wife and friends, enjoying visiting the sights and hearing the sounds of that excellent city, and becoming stronger with each passing day. However, my optimism that this would be the end of my recent acquaintanceship with medical matters and venues was to be short-lived.

On the last day of January 2019 I enjoyed an excellent lunch with a small group of friends at the Betjeman Arms pub at St Pancras Station, feeling that things were going well. A bottle of Kiwi sauvignon was quaffed, celebrating the fact that I had recently returned, with wife Sheila, from the Christmas trip to New Zealand to catch up with son, Steeven, his wife Nicole and infant granddaughter, Georgia.

But the next day I not only spotted signs of blood in my urine, but also found I was needing/having to urinate more frequently. Perhaps I had cystitis. Whether as a result of preparatory tests for the gallbladder operation, or my own subsequent apprehension at noticing intermittent discolouration in my urine, I had recently taken my concerns to my GP, who had initially sounded confident that there wasn't anything drastically wrong, but had reacted very quickly when a PSA blood test result revealed a concerning level in the 40s, and sent me off for a sequence of investigations, each of which seemed to lead seamlessly to another, even though I was still regularly advised that I shouldn't be overly concerned. These investigations incorporated procedures I had never in my wildest dreams expected to experience.

Notably: Twice having a camera inserted down into my penis. Three, maybe four times (I gave up counting) having a finger – someone else's – inserted into my rectum. Undergoing a prostate biopsy, as well as the 'insertion' of fiduciary pellets, when I had been anticipating only a chat with a medic. And during the latter intervention, an unexpected request from a nurse to: 'Please hold your testicles out of the way.'

I submitted docilely to each successive experience – 'Just pop your legs up into these stirrups', 'Lay down and relax while I...', 'Now, this shouldn't feel too...' – actually, almost enjoying them as potential anecdote fodder to some extent, once I'd rapidly realised that the most important element of this probably lengthy situation was to park one's dignity firmly at the door and just do what I was asked, without objection and without really knowing why it was happening.

When subsequent body mining had made it obvious that I was indeed suffering from prostate cancer, it was equally obvious that I didn't have much of a clue what that really meant. Once I accepted that I did have PC, and that it almost certainly wasn't going to go away, I decided that, without having much choice in the matter, I'd better go along with the advice given and the treatment offered. At this point I hadn't told anyone, other than Sheila, what was going on. Should I survive, I vowed to tell family and friends precisely what had happened and how I'd coped – preferably in technicolour detail.

I wanted to be able to tell them about my experiences and to warn the men to get themselves checked out on a regular basis, in case they might be at risk of following the same path with, possibly, a worse outcome. I wanted to do so, using my own experiences as first-hand evidence, and to be able to put into their own minds the possibility that they too might have to travel the same route at some point, and to be aware, I hoped, that it needn't necessarily result in a literal dead end.

I'd heard and read stories about celebrities who had suffered from PC and survived – Rod Stewart, Stephen Fry, Elvis Costello, Robert De Niro, Harry Belafonte, Roger Moore, Ian McKellen and Bill Turnbull amongst them. Golfer Arnold Palmer even founded the Arnold Palmer Prostate Center following his diagnosis. But few of these celebrities' comments and little of their media coverage delved in any detail into what such a diagnosis meant for the recipient. Odd that almost all of them (maybe Mr T gets an honourable exemption), people usually so keen to publicise their every move, change their tune when they are unwell and during their treatments.

I decided to tell of my path to diagnosis in detail, what goes on during treatment, of any potential 'cure' and all that would happen to me along the route. Of the people in similar and worse positions that I met and bonded with during the hours spent being given the significant doses of radiotherapy I underwent – which also meant that I would have to drink an alarming amount of water during the process. In my case, with two buses and a Tube train to negotiate, followed by a dash for home, all with a bursting bladder, this required no insignificant planning in order to ensure I arrived home with still-dry trousers...

Before we really get into this story, though – although I don't want to come across as an unreconstructed pessimist – I have to say I just cannot accept that anyone can actually 'battle' against cancer. I certainly didn't. I endured it, for sure. Lived with it, yes. Came to terms with it, possibly. Worried about it. Stressed out over it. Wondered about it. Confronted it, even. All of those things.

But battled, fought, struggled against it, took it on? No, I don't think so. I don't see how one can. You just submit yourself to the steps the doctors tell you are necessary to give yourself a chance of surviving, even though this will ultimately mean living with what has already happened to you once, and could easily return to do so again.

I'm also not that sure you can ever actually 'beat' cancer. You might be told that your treatment has done what it set out to do, and that, as of now, all of the indications are that you are no longer a cancer patient. But, as far as I have understood things, such a verdict can never guarantee that it can't return, or that you won't find yourself affected by another variant of the disease.

Support for this point of view emerged from an unexpected source in December 2020 when former *Woman's Hour* presenter Jenni Murray appeared in an ITV programme called *The Real Full Monty On Ice*, in which she joined other celebrities promoting cancer charities by stripping on ice live. Jenni, who had had a mastectomy for breast cancer in 2007, declared: 'You don't battle cancer, or fight it, or beat it. You have it and you get on with it.'

TV presenter Bill Turnbull, who has PC, observed: 'You can't fight cancer, you just have to deal with it...' They were both absolutely spot on.

4

IN WHICH I RECEIVE A SPICY WELCOME TO LA

I WAS scheduled to begin the first of 20 radiotherapy treatments, intended to reduce my PSA levels, on Monday 4 February 4 2019. But for the preceding few days the frequency with which I was needing to pass water was definitely increasing. Over the weekend I was seeing blood in my urine and I began getting up two or three times each night to go. Perhaps I had cystitis again? Or it could just be a reaction to those fiducial markers, I supposed. That, and the fact that the need to remain well hydrated, drinking two litres of liquid per day, was obviously going to increase the frequency of going.

But I really wasn't happy about the visibility of blood. So I forfeited a Saturday night out and on Sunday went online to book a GP appointment for Tuesday morning, even though I should by then have begun my radiotherapy treatment and could have perhaps asked then whether this was something or nothing.

Regarding my first radiotherapy appointment I had no idea whether I should report for duty with a full or depleted bladder. I'd previously been up with a group of around a dozen or so other imminent patients to be given a bit of a tour of facilities and an indication of what would happen when and how. I'd also been called in to have a CT scan, prior to which I was asked to drink half a dozen cups of water. I'd later learn (if I had understood correctly), that this was something of a dummy run, designed to reveal certain items of information which would be used to assess the conduct of the daily radiotherapy appointments.

My route to Mount Vernon was not that difficult. Starting with the H12 to Pinner Green. I'd gambled that I had time to visit the post office before catching the bus but as I exited from sending off a package, into the rain, there was the arriving H12. Could I shift quickly enough to catch it? I jogged towards the bus stop, waving like a demented windmill. Not only did the driver see me, he reopened the closed doors to let me on.

At Pinner Green, a brief wait for the H11 straight to Mt V, a mere hour and a quarter early. As I walked damply towards my fate I spotted an on-site charity shop, and bought a David Bowie CD for four bob, surely a good omen for today's adventure.

I used the new-fangled, now soggy, check-in ticket I'd been given, which showed that I had been allocated 'Machine LA 10_2018' at noon. Up came confirmation that I was now to report to LA3 at 12.05. Not a major inconvenience, timewise, but it transpired that LA3 was the only machine without a dedicated waiting room.

I was told to sit in the dimly lit general waiting room and, well, yes, wait for a call. Oh well, I thought, it will be quite interesting to sit amongst the masses who know more about the procedure than a newbie like me.

In such situations I usually prefer to look for a corner position to gaze out at others from, rather than be one at whom others are gazing. Instead, I told myself that as I was about to commence an altogether alien experience it might not be a bad idea to take notes and to begin a treatment diary.

I soon heard patients who were clearly already old hands at this business, chatting about their individual thoughts. Some were complaining about how tired their treatment made them. It was also immediately evident that there were a wide range of complaints and illnesses being treated here, but, crucially, we were all in 'it', whatever 'it' might be for each specific one of us, together.

Said the wife of one patient: 'The other night we were sitting up at 2 am watching the Men Behaving Badly Christmas Special from 1980-something.' Desperation tactics, indeed.

I heard grumbles about the difficulties of accessing the confusing reduced car parking facility for cancer patients. Others were talking about breakfast. I'd had a very early morning slice of toast followed by half a bowl of cereal... I wasn't sure whether this might leave me feeling weak after the treatment. Well, I thought, I'll soon find out.

Steam was rising from damp raincoats, wet footwear and, in my case, a dripping brolly and leather hat, which were slowly drying off, as the packed room held a good number of people waiting for appointments for consultations, follow-ups and treatments.

I noticed a small café dispensing hot drinks, sandwiches, rolls, biscuits and crisps, all at very reasonable prices. Trade was brisk at just after 11am. My gallbladder-free stomach began to rumble a little.

The majority of patients were looking at their mobile phones. Notices on the wall warned against using mobile phones. Being an obedient lad, I'd turned mine off and put it away. I waited in vain for anyone to discipline the illegal users.

A nurse chatted to a handyman who had arrived in the room carrying a step ladder, telling him: 'The poor patients are complaining because it's so dark in here – and if they're not, they're complaining because it's so cold.' She turned and addressed the crowd: 'I'm after two young men...' There were one or two sniggers as the two she was after revealed themselves and she took them away. Who knows where to?

Then I was called for and taken into a room, to be told: 'Empty your bladder.' I had to ask where. Having complied, I was then asked to empty some more to provide a sample, after revealing that I had been seeing blood in my urine sporadically over the weekend. Of course, I could no longer go, having previously done so. So, I had to drink some water to help produce the goods. A charming nurse was fussing over me as a result. A couple of glasses of ice-cold water finally provided a successful conclusion as I silently told myself, 'It makes a change for you not to be taking the piss, but giving it, instead.'

It was tempting to believe that this chain of events was some kind of daily comic sketch laid on for the benefit of newbie patients to calm their nerves. A man walked up to the radiotherapy coffee bar 'Managed by Comforts Fund Charity' counter, holding two empty bottles, and asked the lady behind the counter to fill them. She appeared to be considering whether to ask him precisely how she should do so. Then the man with the step ladder wandered back in, without actually mounting it or appearing to serve any particular purpose. At this point, a man looking rather closer to death's door than anyone else in the room was wheeled through on a bed, on his way to who knows where... Now a guy dressed like a refugee from a hippie music festival sashayed in, somewhat spoiling the grand entrance by dropping a packet of tissues on the floor.

I'd no idea whatsoever how long it might take to run a check on a urine sample, but I began to worry a little when no one came to tell me it was time to drink the six glasses of water I'd been informed were required. Earlier on I had, though, been warned things were running a little late. But what constituted 'a little'? I turned my attention to thinking about the birthday trip to San Francisco I'd booked for my wife and me, knowing that it was one of her ambitions to visit the famously bridged city. I'd been told that the after-effects of my treatment should be over in seven – or so – weeks after it had finished. Which should, I was hoping, just about meet the date we were due to travel.

Suddenly I heard the café lady ask a customer: 'Where are you from?'

'Ware.'

'Yes, where?'

'No, Ware...'

'Nowhere?'

'... in Hertfordshire.'

The café lady told her colleague that people were buying her cakes and sandwiches to take home with them. Cost or taste, I wondered? I hadn't yet sampled them for myself. With tea, coffee, Bovril at 90p, bun/butter for £1, crisps 70p, Cheddars 80p, cake £1, milk 35p, soup 80p, hot chocolate 90p, toast 30p per slice, we're spoiled for choice. Even better, food hygiene rating: 5 out of 5.

The chatty nurse asked a lady what colour she intended to dye her hair.

'Violet.'

No one stayed anonymous for long in there, as various people wandered in with clipboards and shouted out to the room in general:

'CROW? Paul Crow...'

'TYSON? Henry Tyson...'

'BITCH!' The nurse didn't seem to be shouting *at* anyone, but...

'Bitch?' she said again.

'BITCH?!' Again, louder... 'Valerie Bitch?'

Ah, yes, here she was – Valerie BEECH, apparently used to the mispronunciation...

'WINDY?' I'll let you guess...

Eventually I was called to drink my six glasses of H_2O. Out into the corridor to find a dispenser. Sounds easy enough, but it turned out not to be the most pleasurable of tasks, and this was Day One. Phew, done. Back to take a pew again, preparing for... whatever. It feels like the water has gone to my head...

A lady is instructing a nurse about how 'faith' is a 'really important' part of her life. She emphasises: 'We keep on going day after day.'

Having been told I'd need a dressing gown in which to receive my treatment, despite not possessing such a thing, I was surprised to then be informed, 'Okay, just keep the top you have on, that'll be fine,' as I was called in to be zapped. I'd removed my shoes and trousers, retaining pants and socks. The lady in charge asked me to confirm my address and date of birth... 'That's *my* birthday, too' she said, adding quickly, 'A different year, though.' We shook hands, two people linked by a random date. What are the odds? Well, obviously, 364 and a bit/1 – the 'bit' included to allow for leap years.

They put me on the machine, just stopping me in time from

lying down the wrong way round. 'Don't move yourself when we move you,' I was warned, a tad confusingly.

There was a senior medic, male, with a colleague, female, there too. Both matter-of-fact but friendly and efficient sounding, as they lined up my 'tattoos' with, I imagined, my fiducial markers.

Ah, yes, the fiducial markers, aka fiduciary pellets. They'd been 'fitted' a while earlier. 'Fired' might be more accurate. That had been, er, an interesting experience. I won't bore/frighten/disgust you with the gory details (which, safe to say, involved some kind of apparatus which reminded me of the steps on a rope ladder up to a trapeze, although I could have been hallucinating at the time), but instead quote from a website which seems to replicate my memorable experience which, once endured, I tried to lose the memory of as quickly as possible! Seriously, though, another example of parking one's dignity and just letting them what knows get on with it:

Fiducial markers are used to help target the radiation at the prostate gland better. They are tiny, smaller than a grain of rice. They are made of pure gold, so the body does not react with them.

Three seeds are injected into the prostate gland by your urologist or sometimes by another physician. The procedure is very similar to a biopsy: you need to do a bowel cleanse with an enema or magnesium citrate beforehand. You need to take preventative antibiotics for a few days, usually starting on the evening before the procedure. You may be given a sedative at the time of the procedure. An intrarectal ultrasound is used to help guide the insertion of the 'needle'.

One advantage of this compared with the biopsy is that there are only three needle pokes instead of twelve!

The three seeds form the corners of a triangle inside the prostate. When the radiation therapist sets you up for treatment each day, they do a scan which shows the marker seed triangle, and they can finely adjust the treatment table position so that the three seeds line up perfectly with where they are supposed to be. This helps the treatment machine "lock in" on your prostate gland. Think of it as GPS for your prostate.

The other great benefit of all this is the anticipation that one day I'll be asked at an airport check-in whether I have anything of value to declare, and be able to admit: 'Yes, three pieces of gold. Would you like to see them?'

As for the 'tattoos'... I'd always vowed I'd never have one on my body, but I ended up with three, courtesy of PC. Only small ones, and they don't feature slogans or represent loved ones, flags, rock stars, or football clubs. They're blue and initially, I was not really sure what they were put in place for, to be honest. Also helping to line up the zapping rays, I guessed. Cancer Research UK know for sure, though, who say:

During your radiotherapy planning session, your radiographer (sometimes called a radiotherapist) might make between 1 to 5 permanent pin point tattoo marks on your skin. For some types of radiotherapy, for example, electron treatments, you won't have tattoo marks.

Your radiographer uses the tattoos to line up the radiotherapy machine for each treatment. This makes sure that they treat exactly the same area each time.

I'm proud of my three, but rarely show them off these days. Anyway, back to me, stretched out awaiting my first dose of radiotherapy...

'That's it. We won't be a minute,' says the medic guy, as he and his sidekick bolt for the door to get outside as fast as their legs can carry them: in well under a minute as it happens. For what seemed like between ten and fifteen minutes I lay passively, with my hands knitted together on my chest, listening and watching, fascinated, as the radiotherapy machine buzzed, clicked and whirred, and its laser shifted around me several times. I couldn't feel much at all, although I imagined I was experiencing some level of warmth being projected into my nether regions.

There was a rather tinny, pop-y style of background music playing which did not appeal to, or comfort, me. Once the machine had stopped and the huge, thick doors of the room reopened, I was swiftly told to dismount and dress before departing from the room.

'How was that?' I was asked by one of the radiotherapists once I'd emerged.

'Absolutely terrible. I'm shell-shocked. If that's what it is going to be like every time, I'm not coming back,' I told her. She looked crestfallen.

'Oh dear, what happened?'

'I had to listen to the bloody Spice Girls in there. If that's going to happen every day, I'm out of here.'

She laughed. 'Oh... you can bring your own music if you like.'

So, in the future, I vowed I would do so.

Setting off home, I quickly realised that finishing the treatment each day was not going to be the most difficult element of the entire experience. Getting home with dry trousers and pristine pants would be.

I'd utilised the facilities before leaving to wait at the bus stop terminus within the hospital where I was going to catch the H11 to head back homewards. But bus was there none to be seen. There was one due. But how long until it arrived? Remnants of the six cups of water were beginning to stir and inform me that they would like to emerge. So, I popped back to liberate some more liquid.

Still no bus when I returned. Looked like traffic problems were to blame. I began to walk, planning to make it to the nearest Tube station at Northwood. I passed a car whose frontage had been staved in, then decided to catch the 282 bus when it came along, which dropped me off at the station, whose platform boasted a red-coated lady walking up and down whilst plucking away at a Jaw harp.

I got off at Pinner where I had to bolt into the gents before emerging to catch the H12 home, speaking sternly to a boisterous schoolboy who tried to queue-jump: 'Oy, you little jerk, I haven't been standing here waiting so that you can jump in front of me, piss off... !' (Before I do just that, I didn't add!) The young lady getting on in front of me thought I was aiming these remarks at her. Awkward.

The next day I had an appointment at my local GP practice for a urine test, before heading back to Mount Vernon for Day Two. I acknowledged a small gesture of kindness by the bus driver to an elderly chap – no, not me – having difficulty in walking and carrying a large shopping bag. The driver generously stopped the bus before the scheduled stop in order to leave him nearer his destination.

I was again in time to drop into the charity shop at the hospital, this time snapping up CDs by veteran pop stars Crispian St Peters and Tommy Roe – 20p each. What do you mean you've never heard of them? 'You Were on My Mind' and 'Pied Piper' were CSP's chartbusters, 'Sheila' and 'Dizzy' were big hits for Mr Roe on both sides of the Atlantic.

I started chatting with the elderly lady (a good two years older than me) behind the counter. Like a verbal game of tennis, we lobbed back and forth the names of forgotten (by all but us) pop stars like Wayne Fontana, to which she countered with Long John Baldry; and Gene Pitney, to whom she retorted with Freddie Garrity. I enjoyed this diversion so much that I forgot to ask for change from the 50p piece I'd handed over, thus boosting the day's profits for them by two bob (younger readers, ask your grandmother!).

Having checked in again, I was soon ensconced opposite the café, in time to hear a heated discussion which featured the phrase: 'She's so competitive – it's just a bloody game!' Rather the point of any game worth playing, surely? I thought.

The café display was somewhat reduced today – no cake or buns to be seen. Yesterday's somewhat under-employed handyman reappeared, minus his step ladder, but plus a colleague. They studied the lights illuminating the waiting rooms. 'That's good, only two bulbs missing,' observed one. 'Just as well. We haven't got any more than that,' replied the other.

The lady from 'where, Ware?' was also back from Warever, revealing to the much younger lady sitting next to her that she'd had a heart attack and hysterectomy – not, I very much hoped, concurrently. At this point my concentration was interrupted by the radiographer telling me, as though she were the starter for a Grand Prix, to 'Start your waters...' Six more cups of, this time room-temperature, H_2O – preferable to the freezing stuff, I'd decided. Before I went, I heard Mrs Ware telling her companion that of the two, the hysterectomy was the more pleasurable experience.

By now I'd taken to encroaching on the 'posher' part of the not-overly-posh (but bloody wonderful, nonetheless) hospital. For 'posher' read 'private', so it was no surprise when I nipped into their section on the excuse of using their water-dispensing machine pre-treatment, to discover I was able to watch a few minutes of *Wanted Down Under*, a daytime TV favourite in which some working class Brits, pretending to fancy moving to Oz or New Zealand, are flown over to one of those two countries, shown loads of houses they can't afford, offered jobs which will pay poorly, then asked to decide what they wish to do. Which is almost invariably – having seen members of their families tearfully begging them not to go (despite probably not having actually seen them for years) – that they will stay home, no doubt to the relief of Kiwis and Aussies everywhere.

A very posh-plus couple were sitting watching the programme. 'We used to play golf every day,' they said, 'when we lived in America.' But now, they confessed, 'not so much'.

I think the posh gent's treatment was coming to an end, either that or he'd upset the chap at reception, who was now telling the posh man that he hoped he wouldn't have to see him again, but wishing him well for the future. While the posh man popped to the gents prior to leaving, his wife confessed to the receptionist that she could smell the treatment he'd had on him when they drove home together in their posh car. She didn't actually say the car was posh, but it seemed an odds-on shot.

On my return to the waiting area, two young ladies were discussing their cancer-treatment hair loss. One pulled out a wig:

'£15.99 on Amazon,' she laughed.

The other – 'I'll be 51 in May' – had paid £72 for hers, albeit 'with a voucher'.

'Yes, I think it's synthetic,' said the £15.99 lady, 'but it looks quite nice on me.'

They then discussed how other wig wearers could possibly pay 'two and a half to three thousand...'

The 50-year-old tried on her friend's wig, brushed it into place and added a hat. 'I look like Kim Kardashian now,' she said, as the pair took selfies of each other, laughing uproariously.

A girl in a bobble hat was sobbing. Her male companion stroked her head. I think she was the one there for treatment.

Much earlier than had happened the day before, I was being pushed and shoved into place on 'the slab'. Tuesday's audio entertainment – I'd forgotten to bring my own – was Robbie Williams' 'Angels', followed by Britney Spears, then Cher, then young-folk stuff, of which I had no recognition factor.

'Don't you have any heavy metal?' I asked a baffled-looking radiotherapist, before quickly re-robing, squeezing out as much as possible of those six cups' worth of water, dashing off to jump on the waiting H11, followed by another short wait for the H12 and finally back indoors – admittedly straight to the bathroom – before my favourite soap, *Doctors*, started at 1.45.

Shock news on Wednesday, 6 February: I was to switch from LA3 to LA10! Promotion or relegation? I had no idea.

Promotion, I guessed, as LA10 had its own waiting room, with two people doing just that when I arrived. One of them, a chap who had driven 40 miles to get here, and the other, a lady from Wembley, who was worried about the driver of the vehicle sent to collect her who kept knocking on the door. 'My dog goes mad if anyone knocks on the door,' she fretted. Yes, but could the dog bring her to LA10? I doubted it.

Almost as soon as I arrived, they asked me to begin drinking. I lost count during the process, so when I got to what I wasn't sure was either the fifth or sixth cup, I decided to swig an additional half, thus knowing I was only either half a cup over or under the required dosage.

I was called for shortly after, and my treatment began 15 minutes 'early'. I had a laugh with the radiographers who again confirmed that they had no objection to me bringing my own CDs in, if I could actually remember to do so, and also because they played me two Phil Collins or Genesis tracks, followed by Bon Jovi's 'Living on a Prayer', the latter of which I said I hoped wasn't their diagnosis of my condition... However, when they finished the session with more Spice Girls, I knew it was definitely time to fight back with my own selections.

I was dismissed, clutching a new dressing gown for future appointments. But I was far from sure if I'd ever use it.

Opting for a slightly different trip home I caught a 282 bus, quickly visited a couple of charity shops in Northwood, then jumped on a passing H11, on which were some elderly (well, by my standards, anyway) ladies who had all been to the same meeting. One was telling the others how much she loved eating fish.

'Can't see your fins yet,' replied another.

I had to almost physically restrain myself from butting in with, 'Sorry, ladies, fins ain't what they used to be.' Fortunately I'd already got my coat...

I realised that the medical experts really hadn't been joshing when they banged on about pelvic floor exercises helping to extend urination intervals, after I had to get up twice overnight to relieve myself. I told myself firmly to start pelving seriously. I'd also read that Pilates can be helpful in that respect, so I thought I might have a chat with my next-door neighbour, Dr Phil, who had been trying to persuade me to join him in his weekly classes.

I struggled to get an empty bladder on Thursday morning, prior to leaving for Mount V. I was allocated LA10 again and was in position bright and early.

Forty-Mile-Each-Way Man was in residence, as was a family of three: the early-middle-aged (hope she doesn't read this if she turns out only to have been 26) female patient with a supportive crutch and her mum and dad. The latter was a former cricket umpire who, it turned out, was listening to a Big Bash cricket match on his radio as we waited.

Her mum handed over a bottle of water to her when she was instructed to start irrigating herself, and then popped outside to the nearby water fountain, similar to the ones we used to have in the playground at primary school in the '50s (1950s, not 1850s, that is), to bring back two more overflowing cups of the stuff.

We all began chatting naturally to each other. When the former umpire became aware that I used to work for a bookmaker, he told a wonderfully dark story about the day in 1996 when Frankie Dettori rode all seven winners at Ascot, almost bankrupting the entire bookmaking industry in the process, as so many of his fans had backed him to do it...

A friend or relative of the former umpire was being taken to hospital in the final stages of his terminal illness, a day or two after Frankie's astonishing feat. 'As he was being lifted into the ambulance for what might well have been the final time, he turned to his watching friends and gave them a thumbs-up, telling them: "Good old Frankie – he's paid for my funeral."'

Our discussion moved on to the recent apprehension of a previously much-loved entertainer in the grounds of a primary school, from which, along with most of the others in the country, he was specifically banned, then on to intriguingly unsolved murders from past years, such as the Jill Dando and Suzi Lamplugh cases. Black comedy was definitely the theme of the afternoon.

As I went out to the corridor to imbibe my six waters – again losing count... Well, you try doing it! – along came a group of future 'newbies' being shown round by the young lady who'd greeted me a couple of days earlier. As she explained to her group what went on in LA10, I said to her: 'You haven't told them the worst news yet, that they could be exposed to torture by Spice Girls in there, whilst clamped to a bed...'

I'd finally remembered to bring a CD of my own along and the radiographers happily emptied out their player and inserted my Rolling Stones' *Greatest Hits* choice, so I was sustained by 'Not Fade Away', whose sentiments I hoped to comply with, before 'I Wanna Be Your Man', 'It's All Over Now' (I hoped not) and 'Satisfaction' kicked in. I lay there, happily, with radioactive rays shooting into my rear end. Bliss.

That evening, possibly aided by my treatment, our team of Sharpes, Hawkers and Browns actually won the monthly quiz night at Harrow Art Centre for only the second time in over three years... with all of my teammates blissfully unaware of my current medical status.

***

Chilly, wet, windy on the way in – and that was just me, let alone the hostile weather. Still, in a way I preferred these type of days, as they meant not having to feel I was missing anything in the 'real world' by being stuck in hospital for hours.

The last day of my debut week arrived, along with a small surprise as the check-in computer revealed that I was on the move again – this time to LA9. Three different machines in the first week. What, if anything at all, could it mean? Particularly as I'd yet to hear anything about the outcome of my urine test on Monday. I was also now wondering how much, if any, of The Beatles' *Magical Mystery Tour* CD that I'd brought along I was likely to get to hear...

Like LA10, but unlike LA3, 9 seemed to be protected and surrounded by massively thick doors, like some kind of nuclear bunker. Yet I and fellow patients have wandered inside these constructions, clad in pants and jumper, but feeling no fear – other than for the Spice Girls.

I hadn't yet been forced, or even asked, to wear the dressing gown I'd been given – the first I recall owning since the age of about six. Perhaps the staff were just happy to tick the box which says they had provided each patient with one of these, to me, baffling garments.

I wondered whether the machines in each of the LA numbers did anything different from each other, or if they all dispensed the same rays at the same strength... It is amazing what we will accept being done to us, without having the slightest idea of the implications, or even wanting to know. But, when all is said and done, there are plenty of reputable websites out there, many of which can explain what is going on... But I had to accept that I didn't really want to know. At least while it was happening, anyway. I could change my mind later on.

A new middle-aged couple – man and woman – enter. There was also a family of three in the room when I arrived.

Then a new male arrival announced jovially: 'Here we are again. Broke down yesterday, this one, didn't it? They've repaired it, though.' That's good, I thought.

Shortly afterwards there came the Forty-Mile-Each-Way Family, having also been redirected. But my other new 'friends', Mr and Mrs Umpire and Crutch Lady were still in LA10, I noticed, as I took a quick walk to check.

As I started my six cups, Mrs Umpire wandered out and sidled over: 'It's all very boring in there today, no one is speaking to anyone else – we're missing you and the other couple, let's hope we're back together on Monday.' I began to realise that some people didn't have to do the daily six-cup ordeal – I didn't know why there was this difference. But I soon found out that Crutch Lady brought her own patented brew to quaff in her own container.

Despite a scheduled time of midday, they'd asked me to start at 11.36 – and I didn't finish until 11.55. Already I was finding that just the thought of having to drink was beginning to deter my body from wanting to go through the experience.

I was called in at almost 12.30. I checked that I could play *Magical Mystery Tour*. Sure, they said, but then had to run off to find a CD player. Then, when they had nudged and edged me into position, they told me they were going out now, but I had to remind them to turn the CD on. It was brilliant listening to these five tracks. I could really concentrate, with no interruptions or distractions, and the time passed quickly without a problem.

Then, I was finished and with five days – one week – of radiotherapy literally under my belt, I had fifteen left to do. I was released back into the community – free for the weekend, without water to have to drink.

The wind was whipping around, alongside the rain pelting down as I set off home, so I caught the damp H11. But as I narrowly missed the homeward H12, I stayed on board and went all the way down into Pinner, heading for Sainsburys, to take a leak, only to find the men's toilet there closed, and the disabled one in use. So, I had to head for Pinner Station – but the toilet there was locked. Aargh!

I came back out through the automatic gates and appealed to the ticket office guy for the key to open it up, which he handed me – but then, although the ticket machine let me back in and I was able to obtain relief, it didn't want to let me back out. Finally, it relented and I could head for the H12 bus, having to break into a canter as it appeared behind me heading for the stop, only to have to speed up to a gallop to make it, then slumping, breathless into a vacant seat. I got in just as the *Doctors* theme tune was beginning. That's a different kind of relief, as I was rapidly falling for the character Valerie Pitman.

First week all over. It hadn't felt too difficult to cope with, save for the daily six playing havoc with my weeing clock. However, we had been warned that the effects of the radiotherapy would be cumulative, so I figured if I was to get side effects that they were likely to kick in properly at the end of the next week.

I'd read that cranberry juice was regarded as worth drinking if suffering from any urinary problems, despite a shortage of any serious scientific evidence to support such a claim. But £1.39 didn't seem too much to pay for trying it.

It was almost certainly coincidental, though, that – having got up three times during the night on Thursday and Friday – after quaffing cranberry on the Saturday, I was able to attend a football match without having to relieve myself at all, for over four hours. And that night my sleep was interrupted only once by the unavoidable impulse to rush downstairs to the bathroom.

With a week down and three to go I was still very conscious that the treatment effects would build along the way, so I was taking nothing for granted and just feeling thankful that the worst side effects I had experienced so far had been a mild, on-and-off nauseous feeling, a sudden strong dislike of aniseed twist, and a desire to return to butter after over a year of scraping Clover and Flora on to my toast during the build-up to my gallbladder op.

But I still had no idea whether I had, or recently had had, cystitis.

5

IN WHICH I START BETTING WITH MYSELF

EN ROUTE to the first appointment of week two, having enjoyed the weekend break (appointments only take place on weekdays), I headed for check-in, noticing in passing a man fumbling with an envelope, taking out a letter and clearly checking where he needed to go. It made me feel like a seasoned campaigner already, and I stopped myself from asking whether he needed help, figuring that he'd get the same morale-boosting sense of achievement as I did when he managed to manoeuvre his way into the system which would take him through the route we all had to travel during our treatment campaigns.

I'd made a mental betting book with myself en route that I was odds-on favourite to return to LA10 today at the start of the second week. I didn't fancy the chances of LA3, but made LA9 my second favourite, and anywhere else a complete outsider.

I placed a hefty bet with myself before I checked in, but on discovering that the second favourite had obliged, it was off down the corridor to LA9's waiting room.

Striding along, I spotted Forty-Mile-Each-Way Family in LA10, while once in LA9 there was Elderly Irishman just entering the vault to be radiated, as a youngish girl prepared to depart, with her companion, who had just finished treatment.

Elderly Irishman's son said 'Good morning' and told me, 'Dad is going in ten minutes ahead of schedule.' 'Result!' I replied, showing PC solidarity.

The only other person waiting, Middle-Aged Lady, said hello and asked what time I was due in. She was up next, she said, and currently on time.

But I had arrived over an hour before my due time and was prepared for a lengthy wait, only suddenly to hear an instruction phrased as a question: 'Will you start your drinking, please?' What's going on? I double-checked the whereabouts of the Elton John CD I'd picked out for today's prone listening, the mighty *Songs from the West Coast*.

I go back a long way with the former Mr Dwight, having (stop me if you've heard this before, as you will have done if you have read my book *Vinyl Countdown*) taken a call from him – then an unknown – in the late '60s when I was a reporter on his local paper, the Harrow Weekly Post, and he rang up, looking for publicity, telling me that his new single, 'Lady Samantha', had been selected as Tony Blackburn's Record of the Week. Unimpressed, I'd fobbed him off on the chief reporter, Bill Kellow, and a story – plus photograph of him and his sidekick/lyricist Bernie Taupin star-jumping together in their local garden – had duly appeared. Elton, clearly impressed, later included a reproduction of the photo in a booklet which came with his *Captain Fantastic* LP.

My drinking was done by 10.59 – my earliest time yet. As I finished, Forty-Mile-Each-Way Man came out and congratulated me on my team's 3-0 win over Wycombe Wanderers at the weekend. It always amazes me the way fellow football team supporters treat each other as though they actually went out on the pitch to play for their chosen side, in my case, Luton Town. Yes, that win meant we were top of the table in League One, and I was appropriately delighted, so I duly accepted the praise as though I'd put the ball in the net for one of the goals.

After gulping down the half a dozen, horrible H_2Os – I was in. Laid on the slab, zapped, Elton-ed and away, well before my scheduled time. The lady in before me reappeared. Before she'd gone in she'd been reading an article in a magazine which she'd torn out for future study – it was about the alleged medical benefits of cannabis. 'It's supposed to be good for cancer – you can get it from Boots,' she told me. A statement capable of several interpretations, I thought. I mean, who would ever consider that it might be possible to get cancer from wellingtons?

One of the radiologists, Hannah, asked me about keeping hydrated. She told me that tea with caffeine can dehydrate – okay, so that's me back on the decaff stuff, then!

I was back home almost before I'd been scheduled to go in for my treatment. Time travel could yet be possible.

***

Next day I was on the H14 early, so when I arrived at the H11 stop and saw an H13 pulling up, I decided to try it out to find out where it overlapped with the 282, which ends up at Mount V: possibly offering another option for getting to the hospital. Turns out the 'meeting point' for the two routes was outside Northwood Hills Station.

Once I arrived there, I considered taking the tube to Northwood, but opted instead to walk over to the bus stop for both the H11 and 282 (hope you're keeping up with this). The former arrived first, and I'm at Mount V at 10.30, discovering that today the pendulum has swung me to LA10.

I'd not been sat there for many minutes before I heard the phrase 'Start your water, please' and looked around to see who it was aimed at: me!

Crikey. Up I went, out to the fountain, and down with the increasingly foul-tasting liquid, and sitting back down before Forty-Mile-Each-Way Man and his wife arrive. They were bearing tales of 'driving all round the world to places we've never heard of, like

Bushey and Rickmansworth' to get here, as a result of 'two cars crashing on the M3', and as a result they 'arrived at the wrong entry to the car park and had to sit and wait. Still, we're here now. An hour late.' Yes, I thought, and now behind me, as I had since leapfrogged them in the queue.

Mr Umpire and entourage then arrived. Mum was pleased to see me and began chatting away – telling me that it had just been reported that England goalkeeper Gordon Banks had died aged 81. For the benefit of non-football followers, I should add that he was, even then, England's former, rather than current, be(g)loved net custodian.

I was then called in – the Foo Fighters began blaring out; the loudest session I'd enjoyed thus far – and when I came out again it was still twenty minutes before I should have gone in. I feared I was going to suffer for this inadvertent queue-jumping at some stage.

I boarded a 282, got off at Northwood, had a look at the too-expensive second-hand LPs in the jewellery-cum-record shop (don't come across those every day, do you...? Well, unless you live and shop in Northwood, that is). A fascinating place: necklaces, rings and jewels upstairs, and a basement full of vinyl of many kinds – new, old, modern and ancient – to which you are escorted by the proprietor should you show an interest. And I did, and continue to do so. Then, though, I spotted an H11 from a distance, which helped me arrive home before my better half returned from a shopping expedition.

Having asked the radiographers that afternoon whether the routine six cups of water counted in terms of keeping oneself hydrated during the day, they admitted they did, but still recommended drinking as much as possible during the rest of the day to combat the ongoing effects of the treatment. So I quaffed quarts of orange squash and crammed down cranberry juice during the afternoon.

***

On the morning of Wednesday, 13 February, I was sharing the H11 with a man carrying a burgundy red suitcase. He was sitting sideways on, fidgeting with it. Then he changed seats. He was clenching and unclenching his fingers. Fiddling with his hair.

All the signs of someone going in for a stay at Mount V, I surmised... correctly, as I found out when we both alighted at the hospital.

'I really love your hat,' said Mrs Umpire (did I mention I was favouring a black leather Kiwi number as headgear?), as she and Mr Umpire and Crutch Girl arrived, telling us they'd had a good trip down the M1 today, to complete our little LA10 squad, which also included Forty-Mile-Each-Way-Couple, and Relatively-Close-To-Luton Man and – as now became obvious as they talked – his daughter. So, apparently, *not* his wife, as I (and probably the rest of the room) had thought.

Luckily for him, Nearly-Luton Man didn't have to undergo the six-cup ordeal, but I was lucky too that day, being 'done' twenty minutes before schedule, to the accompaniment of wailing albino blues guitarist Johnny Winter, as once again I benefited from the travel travails of my companions from farther flung places.

'Why...' I asked my good lady-wife the next day, as I handed over a card and small box of red paper-covered, heart-shaped chocolates, '...are the initials of Valentine's Day so inappropriate?' She had no answer, but I probably compounded the awkwardness of the moment as, in an uncharacteristic outburst of emotion, I declared: 'I love you EVERY day and not just the one when I am duty bound to do so.'

I wasn't dispensing flowers, and I genuinely dislike the commercialism of this artificial 'occasion', but I can see how others appreciate the opportunity of being permitted, on one particular day by the world at large, to express their feelings without having to worry about being pilloried, pitied or panicked.

Walking in to Mount V and preparing to clock in, I heard, 'Have you finished already?' and looked up to see Almost-Luton Man.

'You must have had a good run down today?' I enquired.

'Yes, and I'm in LA12 today.'

I'd been allocated LA10 again, which meant I'd set a new personal record for consecutive days in one number – this being the third straight occasion. Strolling down to my now familiar abode, I noticed Not-Quite-Luton Man standing in the corridor by the packed LA12 waiting room, looking a little ill at ease and obviously feeling like the outsider that he looked. There were three patients already sat around in LA10. Hmm. Not likely to get away early today, then. One of the waiting guys was asked to 'empty and change', while another rose and with a cheery 'See ya', picked up his gear and departed. The stranger sitting next to me was tapping and shuffling in his seat – a nervous first-timer, perhaps?

When I was called upon to water, I was also told, 'Come on down to LA9 when you're finished.' Sounds like I'm to be a gatecrasher, I thought, as I struggled with the water intake and tried to vary things by mixing ice-cold with room-temp, to no appreciable benefit.

Down in LA9 I sat next to an elderly Irish chap and his daughter. 'I'm 82,' he told me, as folk of that advanced age tend to do, it seems. Mind you, a few minutes later he was revising that: 'I'm 81.' Whatever. He was on the last day of two weeks of treatment having had a cancerous growth removed from the side of his forehead. He'd been told to be very careful when going out in the sun. He used to be a caddy when he was younger, and played golf, too, so he reckoned he'd subjected himself to too much sun, although most of this work had taken place in Ireland.

'Now,' said his daughter, 'he needs a hat – and is mightily impressed with yours. Where can he get one?' Today I was no longer sporting the leather titfer, but had brought my brown trilby – a present from mother-in-law some considerable time ago. 'Debenhams,' I told her.

I was called in for my session, giving the obscure CD, featuring very shrill, very loud '60s guitaring from little-known band SRC, an outing in these rapidly-becoming-familiar surroundings.

Sent off home, I spotted an H11 revving up to depart, which it did, despite my sprint in that direction, definitely putting myself into rear-view and wing mirror visibility in the process, but to no avail. I hurled a throaty 'BASTARD!' towards the uncaring driver and resigned myself to a wait for the 282. It was a beautifully sunny afternoon, so that was no hardship – nor, at that moment, was my bladder, from which I had just managed to empty a good part of the six cups I so recently ingested. No real toilet panic just then.

***

The buses were early enough to get me to Mount V before 10.30 on Friday, 15, the date marking the halfway point in my scheduled treatment. I signed in for LA10 and went there straight away, only to be turfed out and pointed towards a new venue, LA12, where I began talking to a couple who'd come here from Ascot.

The male half had a job involving clearing hospital waste, and told me the amount of apparently still usable equipment thrown away was 'scandalous'. Appropriately enough, we then discussed the episode of *Hospital* on the TV the previous evening in which an 81-year-old from Wales was being denied treatment she'd have had as a matter of course if she had lived in England.

Then I was called upon to do my wearisome water drinking. This time I discussed the process with another chap who had just emerged from LA10 to do the same: 'I've taken to drinking it down as fast as possible.' Indeed, he had. He started behind me and finished in front. Food – or liquid? – for thought.

Having anticipated LA10, then been sent to LA12, I was dispatched to LA3 – 'They can see you quicker than we can.' But when I arrived, it was to shock news – there was no CD player available!

The radiographers were keen to discuss hydration with me and suggested I should be drinking three litres a day – fortunately, that did actually include the six cups, thus, er, watering down the ordeal a little. They advised that at home I should drink squash rather than juice. So, once returned, I headed for Morrisons and invested in two bottles of squash – some sort of orange/mango/passion fruit concoction, together with an apple/blackcurrant combo.

Getting home had been interrupted by a rapid dash to use the facilities at Northwood Station. Relief was short-lived, though, as I had to do the same two stops down the line at Pinner Station, too. I then waited for an H12 which took me to the bottom of my road, from where I had to gallop and push gently past my wife to make it to the bathroom safely.

I received a letter telling me it was time to undergo the two-yearly bowel cancer check. I rang to ask whether my current treatment would present any kind of problem with this, and was told to wait for eight weeks after the treatment had finished before doing the necessary. Those of you who have not had the pleasure of undergoing the bowel cancer check should be aware that it is a painless but somewhat ungainly exercise which also comes under the heading of 'leaving one's dignity at the (bathroom) door', as do so many vital medical practices.

6

IN WHICH I DISAGREE WITH SOMEONE WANTING TO RING THE CHANGES... or IN WHICH I DEAL WITH A DING-DONG

I'D FINISHED my treatment by the time I came across what to me was an astonishingly offensive story, reported on 18 September 2019 by the *Times*: 'A hospital has removed a bell rung by cancer patients to celebrate the end of treatment over concerns that it upsets other sufferers.'

Just let the implications of that sentence sink in. Particularly if you have ever undergone a period of unpleasant but vital medical treatment, after which you have felt relieved and delighted it was over, but are still well aware that there are others just about to start a similar ordeal, or working their way through one. You surely, automatically, wish them well... or do you...?

'The Lingen Davies Centre at Royal Shrewsbury Hospital has taken away the bell after complaints from patients who were unable to complete treatment.' Seriously? Yes, apparently.

Okay, so on that basis: should supporters never cheer when their team scores in case it irritates opposition fans? How would stopping a small celebration of the completion of treatment upset anyone who had not achieved the same? Would it make them feel better to know that they had spoiled a significant accomplishment for someone else?

Some two hundred hospitals in Britain reportedly hold such small ceremonies when chemo or radiotherapy sessions are completed. It didn't happen at Mount V when I finished my radiotherapy treatments, but everyone was congratulatory to me, both staff (obviously keen to escort me off the premises after so many sessions all accompanied by, to them, incomprehensible music) and other patients (clearly had enough of my hat collection and diary writing). I wished them all success with their own treatments and left the building.

Ringing a bell at the end of chemotherapy or radiotherapy has become something of a ritual in some hospitals and clinics around the country. Friends, family and medical staff clap and cheer and the patient reads a poem before sounding the bell to show the disease is in remission.

These ceremonies, often shared by patients online, had inevitably begun in America. I looked for further information about this situation, and discovered a story in the *Shropshire Star*, which told me that a 50-year-old, Jo Taylor, who had been diagnosed with cancer in 2007 and undergone over 80 rounds of chemotherapy, had called for the scrapping of the bell ceremony. She had also founded the campaign group After Breast Cancer Diagnosis, and, writing in the *British Medical Journal*, had declared that it had become a 'modern-day phenomenon' to celebrate 'loudly and brashly'. She said: 'For those of us living with recurrent cancer who have little prospect of being cured, hearing this bell being rung is like a kick in the teeth.' She added: 'People think it's an encouraging thing to have a bell. I disagree, I think it's divisive and cruel. For me, it just reminds me of my own mortality and that I will never get to ring it because I will never finish treatment.'

Tommy Ellis, of Formby, Merseyside, wrote to the *Times* to declare himself 'shocked by the attitude of patients with hard-to-treat cancers who have persuaded the Royal Shrewsbury to remove the bell'. Tommy, who had undergone cancer treatment at the Christie Hospital in Manchester, found the bell-ringing a 'positive and uplifting experience', adding: 'I do not know if my therapy will work but cannot think of any reason why I would want to deny fellow patients, young and old, the chance to ring out in celebration, defiance and in the hope of "beating" cancer.'

His view was endorsed by Gill Mallon on the *Metro*'s website: 'As someone who treasured ringing the bell that signals the end of cancer treatment I was sad to hear that the Royal Shrewsbury has decided to stop the practice. The idea of ringing that bell was the light at the end of a very long tunnel for me.'

In a June 2019 blog, Jo Taylor explained her point of view:

I believe this new way of celebrating finishing chemotherapy arrived from the USA. These bells are generally like a ship's bell or a school bell. They are either mounted on the wall, usually with a rainbow to signify that patients are now at the end of the rainbow and have the pot of gold, i.e. health, recovery, and being 'cancer free'. Or they are like a school bell that you pick up and ring. It is either bought by the hospital ward using donations or patients buy the bell...

I heard it rung three times last week. I sat and videoed my foot nervously waggling as I do when something is on my mind.

Many patients who have been newly diagnosed with breast cancer and are undergoing potentially curative treatment have no idea that overtly celebrating the end of their treatment in this way is so profoundly upsetting for other fellow patients. Modern science has helped many of us to live longer, but in the case of breast cancer there is a risk of recurrence. We know that of those early-stage primary patients approximately 30% will 'at some point' develop secondary breast cancer and that risk can be up to 20 years for some types of breast cancer.

There was no bell to be rung at Mount V and if I'm honest I'm not entirely sure whether I would have rung it at the end of my treatment. But, I am by nature a pessimist. I am not deaf to the feelings of others, and if I've learned anything from my own experience it is that we are all individuals in how we cope with the hand we have been dealt, and should be free to express our feelings in whatever way we wish, provided we are not directly mocking or deliberately upsetting anyone in a similar position. I managed to contact Jo Taylor and asked her to explain her thoughts directly to me:

So no, I'm not in favour but when I had a course of radiotherapy and my two children came with me, they asked me to ring the bell... I did, and immediately cried, as I knew what it meant, but they didn't understand. Children don't, necessarily, do they... ? I've not changed my mind at all – I don't like the bell – it's brash and too in your face and doesn't respect those who have an incurable and terminal illness...

I appeared on *This Morning* last year, and they 'pitted' me against a woman whose child wanted to ring the bell, so that was rather odd – her telling me how wonderful it was, and her child got through because the bell helped him focus – well, if there isn't one there they have to get through anyway. It made me wonder how parents with terminal children must feel heartbroken to see their child die and see jubilant children ring the bell.

I'm just writing a blog about prevention of (breast) cancer (i.e. you can't prevent it...) and I have added a short piece about a child who went to radiotherapy with his mum – she had terminal stage four lung cancer and had palliative radiotherapy... she rang the bell for her child. She later died and the child was traumatised and said 'but she rang the bell'.

If that doesn't make someone stop using this stupid bell ringing, I don't know what will.

I absolutely could not agree with this sentiment. Stopping others celebrating will not improve anyone else's chances of surviving the disease. I cannot imagine that anyone finishing their own treatment would in any way demean or insult anyone still undergoing theirs.

I can understand Jo's despair at her own situation, but criticising and demonising others will surely make not one whit of difference to that situation.

7

IN WHICH I AVOID TELLING MY BEST MATE WHAT'S GOING ON...

THIS DAY – Monday, 18 February – I literally had to stop the traffic – by the simple expedient of striding into the middle of it, arm imperiously held up – to make sure I got across the road and didn't miss the bus, which was arriving at a rate of knots and earlier than scheduled at my stop. I'd forgotten the schools were on half term, which was clearly why the roads were full of fast-moving traffic.

Once arrived I was assigned – as so often before – to LA10. I was scheduled for a meeting with the clinical radiographer, but whether that would take place before, during or after normal treatment, I had not the slightest idea. I only vaguely recognised the two chaps already sat in the waiting room, one of whom was being asked by a female companion: 'How did you get on with your water?'

'Fine,' he answers.

'How long ago did you finish?'

He smiles and says: 'Ten minutes.'

She went off. He collapsed into a chair, head in hands, eyes tightly shut.

Maybe not so fine, then, I thought, but kept my opinion to myself, despite empathising, as it did seem to have become a little tougher for me, too, if I was honest. Mind you, it could have been his first experience, as I didn't recall seeing him previously.

'I think you just get into a pattern... nothing's going to affect me. I'm alright. Then... cancer!' The petite, vibrant lady wearing a red tracksuit top, who I'd first met the week before, was off to start her water. She'd swept in, sat down and begun talking: 'Just this week and four days of next and then I'm finished. It's dreary out there, isn't it?' 'Oh,' she said, looking at me, 'you're reading a book – I wish I'd thought of bringing one. Oh, well, I'll look at the pictures in this magazine instead.'

The other woman in the room said absolutely nothing during this torrent of verbosity, just looked at her fellow female and again said nothing, which was actually a huge relief as she'd been speaking loudly into her phone for the last 15 minutes, despite the obvious bad vibes and looks of displeasure I had been transmitting in her direction... at which point one of the radiographers came in and asked her: 'Can you change, please?'

'No chance,' I thought.

When my three Umpire Family friends turned up it seemed that we were suddenly on informal terms, as they dropped their names – Pat (mum) and Sally (daughter) – into the wide-ranging conversation covering the things that can, but won't, if you're careful, kill you in Australia – with Steve Irwin being held up as the prime example of an entirely avoidable demise, had proper precautions been observed.

I didn't get to queue-jump this time, but at least I was able to listen to Roxy Music as LA10 was, happily, boasting a functioning

CD player. Afterwards, I was expecting to have the treatment review as promised and hand-written on my appointment sheet, but after a short wait I was told it wouldn't be happening on this day.

When I got home – dry, as you ask – I'd received a letter telling me that I would now be receiving a telephone call on 11 April for the review.

It felt good to know I was now 55% of the way through the treatment.

***

Tuesday saw me once again in LA10. A chap I hadn't come across before – bald, wearing white trainers – was told to start his water, whereupon he produced a container full of some kind of liquid, which was definitely not just water... The wrong colour, for starters.

I asked: 'Is that some kind of special brew?'

'Blackcurrant,' he claimed. 'That water is disgusting.' I had to agree and thought this might be a strategy worth borrowing, going forward. I'd bring my own special brew tomorrow, I thought.

Meanwhile, as we'd been chatting, the previous occupant of the room within had emerged, clad in a dressing gown, and been told to 'walk around a bit'. I looked at Baldy, he at me. No words passed between us but we were clearly both wondering what mysterious magic might be going on here? Perhaps he'd turned down the music they were playing and walked out?

No explanation was forthcoming, but a lady popped her head round the door to tell us that 'the trolley' was outside, featuring, she added, a stock of 'newspapers, crisps and similar snacks'. No one was up for purchasing, however.

Baldy was hoping for an early session, as he used hospital transport to get to and from Mount V and it could, he explained, mean a wait of up to three hours after treatment as sometimes the drivers tried to pair patients up, so that one could be dropped off en route to the ultimate location of the other. Baldy needed to get to Welwyn Garden City.

At least my own transport arrangements were straightforward and not so lengthy. Although, that morning, strange rogue traffic lights had appeared, causing significant queues with, as usual, no workers in sight once negotiated.

I asked the Hairless One how many sessions he had remaining. 'Twenty – I've got to have an operation. I didn't know anything about that initially, until they sprang it on me. Brachytherapy, they call it. Thanks a lot, I said!'

This was a startling and somewhat unsettling revelation. However, light relief was at hand as the Umpire Family were now in situ, and squabbling – Sally had accused Pat of wearing brand new shoes, but Pat insisted they had previously been worn, although admitted that since retiring she has more shoes than strictly necessary. The pair then ran us onlookers through the range of diseases and problems each member of their extended family was dealing with. Mr Umpire was, as usual, earplug-ed up, listening to a cricket match taking place somewhere in the world. I tried asking him 'Howzat?' with an innocent expression, but reaction came there none.

Red tracksuit-ed Mary, as I'd discovered she was named – a cheery, funny lady – revealed that she intended to 'get rid of' all the clothes she was and had been wearing during the course of her treatment – evidently wishing to divest herself of not only her disease, but also everything associated with it. Understandable, I thought.

Mr Umpire told us some alarming stories as he revealed – we'd all been too polite to ask – that he was partially sighted. We'd registered the tinted glasses and a stick, but the latter was not white enough to convince us that he was blind. 'It is confusing to people, and sometimes dangerous for me,' he confided, telling us that he had once started heading across a pedestrian crossing only to walk slap bang into the side of a car, which had come to a halt across it, and on another occasion was hit by a non-stopping bus.

I shared a chat round the water-not-so-cooler with Baldy, in which we bonded over our loathing of the taste of Mount V liquid. I really think, I thought, I'm going to bring squash tomorrow. I was in for treatment, and out by the bus stop again a minute after I should have gone in, having enjoyed the session to the accompaniment of the Moody Blues – hardly a night in white satin, though.

***

On Wednesday, 20 February I decided to bring water pre-mixed with orange squash in an effort to minimise the daily drinking trauma.

I set off a little early because of a detour due to affect my route, and ended up using an unusual combination of buses, Tube trains, public toilets and a hearty walk to make it to Mount V.

Once in LA10, one of our 'regulars', who had let slip that he lived in the grounds of a hotel, also revealed that his name was Barry. He was in a talkative mood, and told us that he had not had to wait an excessive amount of time for his transport home yesterday, but that his driver had insisted on following the instructions of his vehicle's satnav, rather than Barry's local knowledge, which resulted in the driver sailing past the road indicated by Barry as the satnav hadn't told him to turn. He then had to make a ten-minute detour to come back to the same point.

'Actually, my postcode suggests that I live in a pub – that really confuses everyone coming to my flat for the first time,' Barry said, who was then called in for treatment a good half hour before his scheduled time.

When it was my turn to start drinking, I had to go looking for plastic cups, none of which were in evidence at the fountain. The machine was only dispensing warm water today, too, so I was relieved to have made up my own mixture beforehand and the added orange squash did seem to make the task slightly more palatable.

When 'Mary' arrived she surprised us all by telling us that she is really 'Marilyn'. She joined in the conversation we'd started on with Mr Umpire and the Umpire Ladies, discussing the 'good old days' and singing the virtues of dripping, tin baths – but not necessarily dripping tin baths – having no central heating in one's house, cutting mouldy bits off of food, etc.

Then we tentatively addressed Brexit. Mr Umpire wasn't a Nigel Farage fan, but did seem to be pro-Brexit and anti-immigration – as was Marilyn. We did, though, somewhat shamefacedly agree that our treatment was probably being provided almost exclusively by second- or third-generation immigrant staff and that it had been unquestionably excellently and expertly carried out.

There was a moment of tension as Marilyn mentioned Muslims. Pat stiffened noticeably and snapped: 'This is offensive. A member of my family is Muslim.' The subject rapidly moved off-limit and we switched to a slightly less divisive subject – ironing.

Later, I struck up a conversation with the substantial gent I'd dubbed White-Beard Biker about an ongoing debate over the future of the Stonehenge site. We both had memories of getting up close and personal with the stones in the '60s.

Having already completed drinking, despite having to search for a stock of plastic cups, I was now called on to undress and prepare. But I was left sitting uncalled for rather longer than had become the norm. I saw one of the medics emerge and talk to a colleague, and, straining my ears, well, lip-reading, really, I was able to make out a comment about the youngish girl who had gone in ahead of me. She had apparently become 'really stressed'.

Eventually, by which time retaining the water I had consumed was becoming a little problematic, I was able to go in and lay down, ready to chill out listening to one of my favourite contemporary blues artists, Robert Cray. Before that could happen we went through the usual routine: the asking of how you've been, then getting you to confirm your date of birth and address to ensure they have the right meat on the slab. Then comes the pulling and pushing to assume the desired position. 'Don't help me when I move you,' they caution. They call out numbers as they move, tweak, nudge and nurdle you into place. Once they pronounce themselves happy, off they go, leaving you completely alone with, you hope, the right CD in the machine at the right volume to entertain you for the next ten minutes to quarter of an hour.

It seemed to be a somewhat longer session than I'd become used to, but once out of the hospital, I not only had to take a slightly different route back than normal, but I also arrived home too late to catch *Doctors*. Later, that evening I feel absolutely knackered – I also think I may have pulled a muscle when taking that quite lengthy walk to the hospital in the morning. And I fancy I'm feeling a bit cold-y, so I slurp down a Lemsip, which often manages to hold off such symptoms.

I was at least still breathing when I woke up on the morning of Thursday, 21 February. The Lemsip had done the business overnight.

As I walked into Mount V to be directed to LA10, I saw Barry walking past me in the other direction: 'Done already – well early!' It was just gone 10.15 am and he looked very happy. I hoped his driver wouldn't prioritise his satnav over Barry's local knowledge on the way back.

Before going into the waiting room I made sure there were drinking cups available to avoid yesterday's shortage – but the stock had been replenished, so no problems there.

I ended up being seen only a few minutes later than scheduled as everyone had turned up on time. I was drinking my squashed water when Marilyn arrived, only a couple of minutes late, but, as ever, looking every inch the rock chick: 'Think I blotted my copybook by mentioning Muslims yesterday,' she smiled, looking totally unrepentant.

So, final day of the week, one week of treatment left after this. But before Mount V I had had to start the day with a hefty wallop in the solar plexus – courtesy of my 9 am appointment with a practice nurse – well, they've had plenty with me...

Nurse Gemma was waiting at my local quack's to administer my tri-monthly Zoladex – a Hormone Replacement Therapy (HRT) – injection. Zoladex, from the AstraZeneca stable (whose Covid jab

I would end up having) works in PC treatment by reducing the amount of testosterone hormone produced by the body. I had had an injection every twelve weeks for some two years, with no noticeable adverse consequences other than an obvious and intended decrease in interest in conjugal relations. Oh, yes, and hot flushes.

She's only running a few minutes late, which is not a problem, and she didn't mess about. She's in good humour and a strong lady, who checks which side she needs to deliver the dosage, before grabbing a couple of fingers' worth of midriff skin, positioning the needle, then whacking the dose in... ...anxious wait... ...but, relief as she confirmed: 'No bleeding.'

Bizarrely enough, Gemma then began an intriguingly unexpected diversion of the conversation – telling me how the windows of the room we were in have now been made 'Peeping-Tom proof', after she'd had a shock once. 'When I was outside and looking over to the window of the room we're in now, with the sun behind me I realised I could see straight into the room.' I told her I would happily volunteer to allow anyone who wanted to, for whatever reason, watch her delivering her best shot to my lower stomach – for a cut of the profits from the TV and internet rights.

Gemma slapped a small plaster over the evidence of her assault on my body – which I knew would soon develop into a small bruise – suggesting that I should now 'relax with a cup of tea'. That idea wouldn't run, but I would, as I spotted a bus heading my way. Burdened as I was by the 'man-bag' – an item I'd always declared I would never own or utilise, until finding a brilliantly designed leather example in New Zealand's capital, Wellington – sitting across my shoulder and bumping the stomach which had just been attacked, I figured there was little hope of my gentle trot getting me to the stop in time, so I waved forlornly in the driver's direction.

Guess what? The driver spotted and waited for me, so I arrived early at Mount V for the final session of Week Three.

I was seriously thinking of giving Barry a new nickname – 'Eight Can Man' – after he boasted that this was the number of beer-filled containers he permitted himself to drink each day. How much liquid each contained was not revealed, and he added that there was an option for more, telling me: 'If I have a drink in the pub I remove one of the eight.' I took that to mean, from his expression, that 'a drink in the pub' might involve rather more than one can's worth, but that only one can would be removed from the non-pub allowance.

Barry offered a tip for helping with the bloated, gassy feelings I was regularly experiencing during the course of forcing down the six cups of water. 'A chap told me to drink half of a Pepsi-Cola first. I tried it – it worked wonders.' So would a Double Diamond, I thought, but didn't say anything. I certainly didn't rush off for a Pepsi, and Barry was uninformative as to whether a Coke would have the same impact.

White-Beard Biker revealed to the room that he was being treated for lung cancer, so didn't have to drink the water as so many of us did. But he'd already had another treatment: 'To be honest, I didn't have much problem with chemotherapy.' Respect.

A day or two earlier we'd crossed in treatment transit – he was coming out as I entered. He'd reached out, touched my arm and said quietly, 'Good luck.' A nice bloke, who was finishing treatment the following week like, I hoped, me.

Bob Dylan's *Together through Life* played while I was being zapped. Not that I didn't like him, but I'd never put Bob at the top of my 'to listen' lists until on a very long flight to New Zealand (there's no other kind, as it happens, at least until Concorde makes a comeback or NZ sensibly votes to move closer to the UK) I accidentally stuck one of his albums on, and then ended up listening to him for several hours – particularly the good-natured *Together* record.

On the H11 bus home I felt a tap on my shoulder and turned round to be told by a very polite young gentleman, probably a quarter of a century younger than me: 'I like your hat. It suits you. Where did you get it from?'

How amazing that this chapeau, purchased for me by a, well, *the* mother-in-law, clearly keen to smarten me up, as a Christmas present, probably twenty-five years earlier, should keep earning me kudos now. 'Suits your face – you've obviously grown into it,' my new friend added. No other item of clothing I've ever worn on any other part of my body, except perhaps one or two of my more expensive leather jackets, have ever earned me complimentary comments, so I was quite touched.

That night, still feeling the HRT injection effects and somewhat fatigued after treatment, Sheila and I went to see and hear the Rollin' Stoned at Wealdstone FC's Tropic club. It was crowded, we had to stand at the back. Halfway through this always-entertaining tribute band's set, I had had enough and we departed.

I spent the weekend regaining some of whatever it was that each week's treatment deprived me of in terms of energy and vigour. I backed a mate's racehorse which was running in this year's renewal of the Eider Chase, at Newcastle, one of their biggest races of the year. West Of The Edge did brilliantly to finish second in 2018. This day he ran as though he'd had to walk from London to Newcastle to take part in the contest and finished a never-threatening 11th. I just hoped that the news filtered through to my owner mate, who was sunning himself on a cruise ship in Miami. That'd put a cloud in front of the sun!

On the Sunday I was at Kenilworth Road to see Luton Town huff and puff to a laboured 1-1 home draw with Coventry. Although it seems counter-intuitive, I didn't manage to stay hydrated for much of the day: perhaps paying the penalty, when overnight I had to get up four times, suffering some stinging sensations whilst producing not very much in the way of urine. I had assumed the daily six-cup ritual during the week would help keep such irritating episodes at bay.

Certainly though, I was not lacking in terms of positivity about the ultimate outcome of my treatment and the very obvious fact that I was far from having to face this ordeal on my own. Friends and family had all been supportive. Although, come to think of it, I hadn't told many friends. Nor family, outside of the closest ones. In fact, I don't think I'd told any of either yet, other than the friends

I'd been making at Mount V, who it seemed to be easier to be frank and honest with as they were in much the same boat.

I had a narrow escape one morning, though, when, striding on to the bus I was confronted by the sight of my oldest chum and his wife sitting there. Somehow, I managed to keep chatting without ever telling them where I was going, and they got off first, without asking me.

8

IN WHICH I BECOME GERRY EMOTIONAL

I WAS not feeling at my best on heading out to catch my buses this particular morning, and was only able to squeeze out a small amount of urine on arrival at the hospital.

In between these two matters I received an unexpected compliment from an elderly lady (probably nearly as old as me) on the H11: 'Noticed your hat as you got on. Very nice.' I was able to return the compliment as she was also chapeau'd. Which gave us both a little mood boost.

I then suffered a minor mental setback, wandering into a very full waiting room in LA10 and finding myself having to apologise as I squeezed into the only vacant seat available and sat down to take stock of this week's patient intake.

Barry had been there since arriving an hour earlier. He had another 14 sessions to complete and seemed to be a 39-er – the number of sessions I had been told is the maximum permitted. I was in for 20, with 15 down already. Barry was pleased to have had a solo ride that morning in his pick-up car. I wasn't paying the attention I should have been, as I was experiencing a gurgling stomach and some uncomfortable, not-quite-empty-bladder sensations.

I'd remembered to pick up a CD for this session in the morning, but now it fell out of my bag while I was fishing my notebook out. The notebook itself had attracted the occasional question, but I'd reassured anyone asking that, of course, I had no interest whatsoever in cataloguing their conversations. Huh! Why would I want to do such a thing?

The sight of the CD prompted Barry to ask, 'Who've you brought along today?'

'Robin Trower.'

'Who's he?'

'Yes, most people ask that. He was the guitarist in Procol Harum back in the day, but then went solo and is probably the closest equivalent to the Jimi Hendrix style of playing still active today – apart from, of course, Hendrix impersonators.' By this time his eyes had glazed over and he really wasn't listening.

The general chat in the waiting room turned to animals. Not in any shape or form a subject which interested, or interests, me. Certainly not since I had my first pet, a budgie called Chippy, when my age was in single figures; nor since my second, a cat, Brooksie – named after my favourite rock chick, Elkie Brooks – died of natural causes; and neither since my third, Tufty, yes, another feline, was ruthlessly run over on her driveway by our next-door neighbour, therefore departing permanently to the great menagerie in the sky. Sheila would love to own a greyhound, and I am not totally against that, but pets undoubtedly adversely affect one's freedom of movement, as well as taking over most of the house for themselves.

I may have mentioned some of this to the rest of the waiting room, but I fell silent when I accidentally found out from clues in the conversation that Mr Umpire is married to Sally – I'd thought he was Pat's partner and Sally's dad. Jumping to conclusions again!

Barry was rather miffed about how long he'd had to wait for his transport home the day before.

Overall it seemed to be an uneventful treatment session, but the day soon turned very eventful...

When I returned home I found that Sheila was unwell. She'd been sick several times – once over the expensively purchased, framed reproduction of her favourite single, 'Tin Soldier,' by the Small Faces, which I'd bought as her Christmas present but which we hadn't yet got round to hanging on the wall.

This was all something of a throwback to many years ago when these sort of symptoms could be commonplace for her: not necessarily alcohol-induced! Nor pregnancy-related... Nonetheless it was a little alarming, until she managed to crawl into bed and go off to sleep. Fortunately, she felt much better the next morning and we put it down to some rogue foodstuff not agreeing with her. But at least it was unlikely to indicate pregnancy.

Now I also had to deal with the email I'd received, telling me that my radiography assessment would happen on 13 March. There was no time given for the meeting, and as I would not be going to the hospital regularly by then I thought I'd better ring and find out when and where it would take place: 'I was wondering what time the review will happen so I can make sure I'm there.'

'Don't worry, we'll come and find you before or after your treatment on the day.'

'But I finish treatment shortly ...'

'No. We have you down for treatment until 28 March.'

'What!? But that's a month away! Today's 26 February. I'm scheduled to finish on 28 *February*.'

I'd been working on the presumption that, having been given an appointment schedule of 20 daily treatments, that would be what I would get. Now, a quick calculation suggested I was actually going to have what was the maximum number of permitted sessions – 39 of them – virtually doubling what I'd been given to understand.

Questions and concerns came flooding in. Was this good, bad, neither? Did it mean they'd discovered I was in a worse position than I'd assumed, or was it just a case of a cock-up rather than a conspiracy?

I'd have to wait until the following day to ask these questions.

Which didn't stop me feeling outraged, annoyed, worried, that no one had officially informed me of my true situation. I managed to rationalise the extra activity. I'd survived pretty much half of the new total amount, so felt confident that if push was going to come to shove, I'd be able to survive the same again. But this was really the first proper setback or problem I'd encountered along the way. Perhaps I'd taken everything too much for granted. Not realised the true gravity of my situation.

Anyway, in light of my earlier Robin Trower explanations, I decided to bring the 'real' Jimi Hendrix along with me for the next day. I now knew I'd have to nominate a further 20 favourite artist(e)s to accompany me through to the end of treatment.

I was slightly late and there was no Barry to be seen, but one of the ladies usually there before me had just gone in. I was done with the watering by 10.51 am – two hours earlier than yesterday – and by now was the only person left in the waiting room. Now I was joined by a tall fellow, bald, or with his hair deliberately cropped so short as to seem so.

'How are you?' he was asked by the radiographer.

'Bit rough.' He answered.

'Yesterday's chemo?'

'Yes.'

He did appear to be struggling. I began to think I might have been treating my own experiences a little lightly when others were clearly suffering traumatic times just because of their treatment, let alone the direct effects of their illness.

Barry finally arrived. His lift had been late, but he wasn't concerned when I suggested I may have been given his time slot as a result.

I chatted to the radiographer, who reassured me that they had always had me down for the 39-session treatment. I wasn't sure I totally believed that, but what difference did it make? I was definitely in for the long haul now, like it or not, so I might as well accept the former version of events. Hendrix was a little jarred by my new situation it seemed, to judge by the way the CD, featuring his greatest hits, was jumping and sticking during playback...

***

On Wednesday morning, 27 February it occurred to me that LA10 was showing signs of becoming a confessional for its regulars.

Barry was in situ and had already done his water. I was then quickly asked to do my own, which I'd decided would go down more easily if I tinted it with the so-called strawberry-flavoured water I'd purchased from Morrisons yesterday – and which tasted positively disgusting. Without it I'm sure I would have finished earlier than 10.31.

When I re-entered LA10, only Barry was there. He began to confess to me that he owed the tax man a considerable amount and that he was effectively fiddling his way to more disability pension than he was strictly entitled to. And he unburdened himself further, possibly a little less interestingly, by adding that he was being regularly 'caught out by wet farts'. We were then joined by Neck-Cancer Man who told us black-humoured tales of projectile vomiting and internal ulcers, related to his chemo course.

Marilyn turned up and soon lightened the tone: 'Are you both prostrate?' she asked.

'No, we can also stand up,' I replied, feeling a gust of wind as the remark jetted straight out over her good-humoured head.

Totally unfazed, Marilyn continued, 'I did some reading up about prostrate and read that men of 50 and over need to ejaculate 25 times.'

'What, a year? A month, week, day – how often?'

'Can't remember.'

At my age, my money was optimistically on *per year*. Before I started on the HRT, that was, anyway – now that might be *per decade*.

Called to get undressed, I entered the dressing room as Barry came out. A new, male radiographer put my CSNY CD on and, as I lay down, preparing for nudging, nurdling, pushing, poking and prodding into place, he looked straight at me, with a serious expression: 'There's only so much we can do for you.' This genuinely shocked me – until he laughed loudly, pointing at the Luton Town FC shirt I was wearing. Then shocked me more by confessing to be a supporter of 'our deadly enemies' Watford FC.

'We do have a radiographer who is the other Luton fan!' he added. I immediately asked for a transfer...

As I re-togged, the chief radiographer turned up and told me that I'd taken longer than usual to do today as I 'had some gas in [my] bowels which caused a slight obstruction'. He gave me a leaflet about such matters and I promptly repaired to the facilities to try to de-gas, largely to protect the good folk I'd be sharing public transport with on the way home. On the way out I received a wave from Mr Umpire and Co who'd been banished to a different waiting room that day.

En route home I was attracting more hat envy: 'You look familiar in that hat – don't tell me, I've got it – J R Ewing.' Can't please all the folk all the time...

Next morning, I guessed it might prove to be a dodgy day when I left the house at 9.30 am, only to see the H12 disappearing round the corner. Then I realised I'd left my phone at home, so thought I'd go back for it.

By the time I emerged from the house again it was 9.52, but a smooth run through got me to the hospital by 10.30 – about the time I'd finished drinking yesterday.

Today a run of 11 straight LA10 appearances was broken as I was dispatched to LA9, which was packed when I arrived, and one of the radiographers was looking harassed whilst attempting to calm down patients who all seemed to be running late. Not a promising sign. Eventually they began to ship people out to other venues, and it wasn't long before the 'dream team', as Pat had dubbed us, was reunited in LA9. Mr Umpire and Sally were in place, but she seemed worried about when she'd be called on to start drinking and was reluctant to go to the toilet in case she lost her place in the queue. We told her to go anyway as none of us had any idea how long we might be waiting.

'But there's no toilet nearby,' she wailed.

'Yes, there is - the disabled one over the corridor.'

'I don't want to use disabled toilets,' said the plainly disabled Sally, whose crutch we had been given to understand was essential, following an accident. 'I don't like them.'

She stayed where she was, and eventually only she, Barry and I were left - with me having the latest scheduled start time, even though by now it was 11.55, which had me thinking I wouldn't be out before 2.30 pm.

Alex, the Chemo Man, had come in with us and was now discussing what he might do with his chemo mask, which he'd been told he could keep. He thought he might put it in his garage. 'On a plinth,' I suggested.

We began discussing the Mexican Day of the Dead, not that anyone seemed to know much about it, or why we had ended up discussing it. There was no Marilyn visible - she'd been shunted off to LA7, we learned from the bush telegraph. Then we discussed whether we were permitted to keep jumpers on during treatment. It seemed to depend on who was in charge at any particular time in the laser room.

Further interesting discussions broke out: how to make chocolate brownies, which of us did or didn't want to know exactly what was happening to us with regards to the intimate details of our treatment. I was in the 'don't tell me, I don't care, just leave it to the experts' camp, joined by Chemo Man. Others wanted to research and discuss their own ideas with the medics. I said that was like all the people who'd only ever popped occasionally into a betting shop wanting to tell me, a veteran of over 40 years in the bookmaking business, about the evils of gambling.

I went out to start drinking. One of the radiographers came over, 'We do feel your pain, having to do that every day,' she sympathised.

En route home I popped down to reception to ask whether they had a lost property department, as I feared I had lost my prescription glasses.

'We don't have a lost property facility as such, but we do keep a few things that have been handed in, but we only have this pair of glasses.'

'Woo-hoo, they're mine!'

'If you can see them from there, you probably don't need glasses!'

Despite the delay that morning, I was able to make up time, and got home shortly after the end of *Doctors*. But I caught up with the episode later that evening, only to be shocked by what was happening to my beloved Valerie Pitman, who had become a murder suspect!

***

As Friday, 1 March dawned, it immediately occurred to me that this may have been my final day's treatment under the original schedule I'd been given. Instead it was merely the halfway point.

Oh well, onwards and upwards. I again drew LA9 and was in there by 10.30, telling the only other occupant, 'It was like Waterloo Station in the rush hour here yesterday.'

Despite having been told that LA10 had been scheduled for a service this day, it seemed to be open for business. My sole companion went out and I was left in not-so-splendid isolation, shorn of my regular pals. I was joined shortly by a difficult-to-understand, grey-haired man, complaining that he'd been moved. 'What's wrong with 10? That's what it says on my schedule,' he asked me, as though I was privy to the daily scheduling of the machines.

It didn't take long to realise my thoughts of an early call were not going to be granted. It was all going tits up.

One of the radiographers came in to make up, sorry, explain, the reason for this morning's late-running schedule as two escapees from LA3 arrived to queue-jump, along with several other characters I'd never met before. There was neither sight nor sound of the Umpire clan, nor of Barry, Chemo Man or Marilyn. I felt alone in a sea of unfamiliar newbies, but settled down behind the pages of *Fortean Times* magazine, seeking anonymity in such strangely unfamiliar surroundings, and worrying that this could be how it would be from here on in.

There was a bright moment when the Quiet Old Boy who had been an unobtrusive and anonymous presence for much of my time there knocked on the glass and waved what was presumably a fond farewell to us. Nice of him.

Suddenly Pat arrived at the door, to tell us that the Umpire Crew were in LA10, and that Sally had had her water – almost certainly meaning she's going to finish before me. 'See you on Monday,' she predicted or promised. I wasn't sure which, but hoped the latter as they'd been very supportive and optimistic, despite every member of their extended families apparently having contracted awful diseases or suffered from terrible accidents. Really like them; wouldn't want to be related to them!

Now I was left in a room of six strangers with no idea when or how I might escape. One of my worst days thus far, despite having expected it to be the best when this adventure began. Very few other 'waterers' brought things with them to read, other than their phones. An occasional one would pick up an abandoned, out of date paper or magazine lying about in the room, but no one ever bought a new one from the trolley. Most people sat in silence. I thought: our little group is something of an outlier, in a sea of silently suffering solitary souls.

A man with a brightly sunburned face – possibly caused by his treatment – arrived amongst us. There followed a sniffling woman and an elderly gent with a young, female companion, probably his daughter. This latter couple were plotting a route to Northwick Park Hospital – just a few miles away and where both of our sons were born – when they were finished at Mount V.

I finally got to imbibe my liquid, but forgot to note the time I'd finished, and started talking to a new Biker Man, who turned out to be a fellow record collector. Of course, I couldn't have known it then, but Ron and I would very soon become great chums.

Then I was asked when I had finished my water and I couldn't remember, but was told I was going to be dispatched elsewhere to an LA where I could be done more quickly... While I waited to hear where the new venue would be, I chatted on to Biker Man, who specialised in 78rpm records, instrumental guitar records, Chet Atkins, Bert Weedon, Jet Harris et al... Then I was told to leg it to LA7: 'It'll be quicker there – they're ready for you.'

Indeed, they were ready for me but – and there was a hefty *but* – the facility lacked a CD player. And there was I, despondent at the thought of missing out on today's brilliant Gerry Rafferty music.

However, one of the – female, young – radiographers showed the other my CD and the latter rushed off, telling me she'd 'Spotify' it for me. No idea what she meant or how she achieved it, but within a very short space of time, the distinctive Rafferty vocals had appeared in the ether. Not the actual album I'd brought with me, but an equally brilliant bunch of songs.

This was one of the most emotional moments I had experienced during the whole process. Such a kind gesture done for someone, by two carers he had never so much as seen before, and whose choice in music almost certainly would have baffled them. They didn't need to do it. I wouldn't have complained had they not. But that they did would stay with me as a key element of what I am determined *not* to refer to as my 'journey'.

I finished the day's activity at about 1.30 pm, and was wished well by a chap emerging from LA7 who told me, 'I've only got one left.' Hearing my 'I've got 19 more' reply, he reached out, shook my hand and added, 'I like the hat.'

I passed Barry on the way out – as ever, waiting for, not Godot, but his next lift. We also shook hands. 'See you next week,' we both said, which would be Barry's final week.

I had to de-water in double-quick time at both Northwood and Pinner Stations: at the latter, persuading the cleaner who was attempting to lock it behind her, to relent. Which, good-humouredly, she did.

Once in Pinner and with no bus in sight, I headed for the bakers and bought a huge jam doughnut. While remembering my last purchase here at Wenzels – current sponsors of the local football team I have supported for over 60 years, Wealdstone – which had been a Chelsea bun, I thought that on Monday, to celebrate moving into the second half of my treatment, I'd opt for a Belgian bun...

9

IN WHICH IT'S RON TO THE RESCUE – ARE YOU SURE?

ALL OF a sudden I began to feel that I needed a new daily routine. This was somewhat discomfiting, having finally managed to put everything in place for the first few weeks when my appointments were all theoretically due to happen at noon, my new schedule was showing a variation of times to report for duty, the earliest being 2.45 pm.

I was concerned that this might mean I'd now lose contact with the familiar friends – as I felt I could already call them – that I'd made over the past four weeks, and have to carve out new relationships with a different band of fellow travellers. So far what I had anticipated might well be a stressful and anxious experience, had been anything but. Now, though, I felt I was about to be taken out of my comfort zone.

My second-half appointment schedule began on 4 March 2019 at 4.40, with a theoretical visit to LA10. I selected the band Supertramp to accompany me into the laser room. Until now my daily objective had been to get home in time to watch *Doctors* if possible, at its 1.45 starting time. Now, I wouldn't be leaving the house until well after that time and, what's more, I realised that even my subconscious was under strain, as I headed out of the door without taking my pre-prepared bottle of chilled water out of the fridge and had to nip back to do so, thus risking missing the bus, although I did make it to the stop in time.

When I arrived at the second bus stop, my text from TfL, or whoever it is that predicts the time of arrival of buses, told me there wouldn't be an H11 for 13 minutes. However, I could see something that not only sounded like an H11, but looked like an H11 and appeared to be travelling along the route of an H11. So I boarded it, and I reached Mount V at 2.50, almost two hours early, but was depressed to see a sign declaring '30-Minute Delay', and a LA10 waiting room packed with the faces of unfamiliar patients. I did, though recognise radiographer Suresh on my way in and he seemed to register mine as a vaguely familiar face. The system seemed at least to be moving, albeit slowly, although a man who arrived, to be asked 'Have you taken your pill?', said he did so at 2 pm, confiding to another member of the waiting room that he had since been walking around for an hour and a half, but gave no indication why.

A lady was called out: 'Follow me.' Her companion wondered how long she might be gone. 'About 15 minutes,' she's told, and I guess she's here for a consultation. Six of us – four male, two female – were now sat together, all solo, I surmised. One checked his watch. A man emerging from the treatment room knocked on the glass and, as one of the ladies acknowledged him he told the room at large, 'Okay, bless you,' which was nice of him, if probably futile. People in here seemed to be on their best behaviour. I'd sat here many times but the atmosphere was now subtly different. Another male patient was asked to 'Start your water' and went off to do so, muttering, 'Half hour late', only to return quickly to pick up his dark green water container.

My mind wandered off. When would I be able to discuss any of this with anyone other than Sheila or my fellow patients? If all progressed as intended, I'd probably still have to wait for a scheduled meeting in May with my consultant to discover how things stood and whether this was just an opening tranche of treatment. By then, I pondered, the football season would be over, Luton would probably have ended up in the play-offs, Wealdstone FC likewise, and my Kiwi team, Wellington Phoenix, might also have fluked a place in the A-League play-offs.

We'd have been to San Francisco, seen Wilko Johnson play a concert at the Alban Arena. Likewise, we'd have seen the Counterfeit Stones. We'd have contested three more monthly quizzes with our team of friends. We may even have had a couple of days down in Brighton or Eastbourne. We'd also be moving close to our highlight of every year – our annual trip to Jersey. Possibly, too, – we'd be planning an August trip to New Zealand to see our two-year-old granddaughter Georgia, her dad – our son Steeven – and her mum – our daughter-in-law – Nicole. I also very much hoped that my current favourite racehorse, Apple's Jade, would have become the Champion Hurdler.

I was awoken from my reverie to hear Suresh calling in a tall gentleman, tapping him on the knee to gain his attention. 'Come with me, sir.'

'You're only calling me "sir" because you've forgotten my name, aren't you?' Suresh neither confirmed nor denied the allegation.

It was now 10 to 4. Since I had walked in no one had spoken, nor addressed any remarks directly to me. A new lady came in, sat down: 'Another week to go,' she said. If only that's all it was...

My appointment was for 4.45, but it was half an hour later than that that I was ascending, not the throne, but the laser target bed, and being overseen by my Watford-supporting medic, and his friendly blonde colleague, who insisted on calling me 'Graham'. This is my name, of course, but given that everyone else called me 'Mr Sharpe', it just felt a little out of sync.

They were both well briefed, and when I handed over the Supertramp CD the female colleague agreed to turn up the volume. 'She's a bit of a rock chick,' said Hornets-Boy.

'The Logical Song' boomed out, probably loud enough for the waiting room to get an earful, too. I was now beginning to worry it may be *too* loud, but there were no complaints. I explained my recent irregular urination problems to the Rock Chick. 'We call it radiation-induced cystitis,' she explained, relatively unconcerned, which reassured me that it was a nuisance, not a problem. Home again by 6.15. I chilled out by sitting with son number two, Paul, to watch Alan Partridge... A-ha...

I only had to get up once overnight, although I had a couple of stomach issues during the day in both morning and afternoon. I wasn't sure whether it would be permissible to take any medication to try to stop the symptoms, as Barry had told me he'd done on a couple of occasions. I did politely tell Sheila that I didn't think it would be a good idea for me to consume the pea soup she had made for lunch, and instead opted for a toasted cheese sandwich and a banana roll which I thought might steady the, er, ship.

***

The next day, I was able to watch a little of the latest episode of *Doctors* before heading off for my 4.35 appointment, which gave me time to have a look into the hospital's excellent charity book shop, where I was able to jog the memories of the elderly volunteers, who were struggling to recall a name temporarily eluding them both: 'Suzanne Dando,' I told them.

Eventually deciding against buying a couple of Spike Milligan books, I joined today's less formal throng in LA10 where yesterday's rather strained atmosphere had been replaced by chatting and joking... as well as the arising of an interesting difference of opinion. When one of our radiotherapists stuck her head round the door and asked a question of one of the gang – who says he is a teacher – he answered: '2.57'. After which she disappeared. The tall chap next to me thought she'd asked him to get changed, as did I. But two others argued that she'd asked what time he'd finished his water. Odd. I decided not to contribute to the conversation, as I would be dropping back in appointment time by nearly two hours tomorrow.

As the founder of, and a judge for, the annual William Hill Sports Book of the Year award, I'd brought a couple of early contenders along with me to check out while I was waiting. The one I began reading was rugby union legend Doddie Weir's autobiography. He was now suffering from motor neurone disease and his insight into how someone, used to physical strength and sporting conflict, deals with a disease threatening medical infirmity, promised to be a fascinating theme.

One of the radiographers came in to ask everyone how they were getting on. I told him I felt like I had jetlag after the switch from morning appointments becoming mid to late afternoons. 'We're running a bit closer to time today,' he claimed.

'Hmm. I'll be the judge of that.' I told him.

He was not far from being right, and after rocking the laser room with a severe blast of AC/DC, I celebrated with a jam doughnut from Wenzels. Overnight I had to get up three times. The doughnut wasn't to blame.

***

On Wednesday, my appointment time was much earlier than at the beginning of the week – 2.45 pm – and I was hoping as a result to spot some familiar faces, and, joy of joys, my new PC/vinyl buddy, Ron, and his charming wife Jan were there. As was the Jehovah's Witness, Dave Dhunna, with whom I – and a number of fellow patients – had recently shared a couple of intriguing conversations. So keen was he to lure some of us into his area of interest that he'd drawn my attention to a 224-page book entitled *What does the Bible really Teach?* and a pamphlet, *Good News from God!*, somewhat shorter at 32 pages.

If I was honest I had zilch interest in what his publications had to say, and even less in the message he sought to bring me about a deity quite happy to deny a blood transfusion to those – even children – who were suffering from terrible, life-threatening diseases. That message basically being, as far as I could understand it: forget it, you'll have to die, if that's the only option.

Anyway, Very Tall Man was also in the room, and he introduced himself as 'John Buchan – but not the novelist'. As another guy exited the room, Very Tall Man called over his shoulder, 'Cheers, Rob.' 'Rob' looked up and corrected him: '*Andy*,' he said, adding, 'We've only been waiting together for three weeks, suppose I can't expect him to remember my name!' Ron, a large, instantly friendly bear of a chap, told me proudly he'd just that morning purchased a 45rpm single by The Allisons from a charity shop in St Albans. I immediately remembered them as the duo who had won the Eurovision Song Contest for the UK, way back in, probably 1960, with their ditty 'Are You Sure?'.

I checked later, and they came second and it was 1961. Whatever. I was 10 and 11 in 1961 and I suspected Ron had been a little older.

The single Ron had bought was called 'Blue Tears'. Not a track I could quite call to mind, but it cost him a mere quid and, oddly enough, he didn't seem to be, er, sure if he knew 'Are You Sure?', their greatest hit. Importantly, though, Ron wanted to exchange phone numbers, something I was positively delighted to agree to. I later discovered how he'd clocked me for the first time, as he'd kept his own diary, which read:

Around this time we'd seen in the waiting room a new face, a chap sitting in the corner, wearing a cowboy hat [Reader – this was me, your author, and I'm here to tell you that that was not a cowboy hat, but a black leather Australian outback hat!] and leather jacket. "Hello, mate, how're y'doing? Everything going well?" I noticed against the leg of his chair a carrier bag with the words "*Fortean Times*" written on it – a kindred spirit, maybe?

We would quickly discover we were indeed kindred spirits.

The afternoon rapidly spiralled into one of the most bizarre of the entire experience. First, Dave, aka Divendra, revealed to the room his experience of eating insects, of visiting the Great Wall of China, of finding a wife in that country and becoming a Jehovah's Witness five years earlier. The younger lad with him was, he told us, a fellow Witness, who had driven him to Mount V. And Dave/

Divendra then told us he was about to start converting the rest of us. Ron was emphatically not up for being converted. John Buchan was emphatically sceptical about what he was being asked to sign up to.

I decided to draw him into a debate, which did, at least for a short while, interrupt Dave/Divendra's flow, as did the instruction: 'Come and get changed!' After which he left, promising to return tomorrow, armed with even more literature. A somewhat stunned silence reigned for some moments after Dave/Divendra went in for his treatment.

Buchan and Dave/Divendra did have one thing in common, though – a list of terrible side-effects from their hormone injections featuring leaking boils, fatigue, excruciating headaches, painful scalps and many more. I felt a little deprived at not yet having experienced (m)any of these, wondering whether they all lay in wait a way down the road...

We all agreed, while sitting around chewing the fat, that we felt like members of a privileged club, sharing our experiences and feelings, of which the outside world knew nothing – or not yet, anyway!

At last, I was sent out to water. Around the fountain were an elderly gent – not quite as doddery as first glance suggested – and a lady up (down?) from LA12. She promptly glugged five cups in very short order indeed, and brazenly but accurately called the two of us 'wusses and wimps' in the process – quite reasonably enough, as I was definitely struggling to quaff mine in similar style – before she dashed back to the sanctuary of LA12.

The Old Boy told me that the day before, he'd been left waiting for his afternoon lift home until 9 pm.

Soon after, while I was being done to a turn to the sweet rock sounds of Wishbone Ash, I was left somewhat 'ash'en-faced when my friendly Watford-fan radiographer informed me that my bladder appeared 'to be three times its usual size' today, and that I should endeavour to empty rather more before commencing in future.

Easier said than done, I thought, whilst nodding and promising to oblige... somehow... Then I headed for home and bought myself a Belgian bun for 95p from Wenzels on the way.

Once indoors, I probably wasn't making it that much easier for my digestive system by forcing down three of the pancakes Sheila had made for Paul and me. Albeit a day late, apparently...

***

I hadn't been looking forward to Ron's last day – well, his last amongst us radiotherapy sessioneers – so I had appropriately opted for a blues CD to mark the occasion, by the Tedeschi Trucks Band. Not that Ron had ever heard of the group, nor been aware of how much pleasurable conversation and atmosphere the departure of this amiable and engaging man and his lovely wife would remove for me from the daily grind of the various LAs we frequented.

Ron wasn't finishing his relationship with Mount V though by any means – his next stage was going to be a three-day stay here the following week, while he underwent brachytherapy treatment. 'Brachytherapy is a form of radiotherapy where a sealed radiation source is placed inside or next to the area requiring treatment. Brachy is Greek for short. Brachytherapy is commonly used as an effective treatment for cervical, prostate, breast, oesophageal and skin cancer and can also be used to treat tumours in many other body sites. The positive news is that multiple long-term brachytherapy studies have found recurrence-free survival rates of 77 to 93%.'

Our resident Jehovah's Witness had been dispatched to a different waiting room. This relieved me of having to pretend to be interested in the reams of propaganda – sorry, fascinating and informative material – which he had promised me. Ron – and this tells you a great deal about the nature of the man – had brought in the 1961 Allisons' single we'd been discussing the other day, just so that I could see, touch and appreciate the longevity of the record. However, when I did get hold of it, a quick shufty showed that the side he had suspected of being the A-side, was in fact the B, so I was able to put him straight on which of the two tracks was expected to make a splash in the charts back then.

Jan was with Ron as ever, but explained that next week a daughter would be drafted in to bring Ron in for his treatment, as Jan is a non-driver. Ron had his own tactics for water drinking – he believed in quaffing bits here and pieces there, only topping up to the full amount when the instruction to imbibe was delivered. It didn't seem to have affected the procedure adversely in any way. We all had plenty of laughs that afternoon, and Ron had also brought with him a flyer advertising a market in St Albans which routinely featured dealers with 'boxes of records'. We agreed that when we were both free of restrictions we would meet up in the Cathedral city.

We both finished our day's lasering. I think Ron went in before me. I don't remember too many details of what was an unexpectedly emotional afternoon, but I got through, with the later assistance from a Wenzels Chelsea bun, which I was enjoying so much that I forgot to look up when the bus came along, and missed not only it... but Ron, too.

***

The next morning I was listening to a 36-year-old (she told us this!) young lady telling me how she lost her hair when she started chemotherapy. Once she knew it was going to happen, she pre-empted that traumatic experience and enlisted her Dad to shave it all off in advance.

She also said she now had 'breasts of differing sizes', and was having radiotherapy to ensure her cancer wouldn't return, although she was 'officially' cancer-free. She had had lymph node removal. She was sparing no intimate detail and suffering no embarrassment in discussing her situation with we three elderly blokes, sitting alongside her in the waiting room and listening very sympathetically, all of us probably thinking, sadly: 'This could be my daughter or niece talking.'

I won't forget that experience. Or that brave lady, who told us that, yes, her hair had grown back, but in a different colour.

An older woman joined our little group. She was accompanying her mother, who had two tumours. 'If you have the strength of mind you can get through this and overcome it,' the younger one told her. I bit my tongue. That's not necessarily true, I thought, but kept my counsel.

When I'd checked in – before I made my way down the now-very-familiar corridors to LA10 – I'd been told that I had an appointment before today's session. This was not something I'd known about in advance, and the news made me a little apprehensive.

A chap came in who I vaguely recognised, and asked me, 'Are you late?' I told him my times had altered from my initial sessions, and he told me he'd been having earlier appointments. Just now he'd had his final one.

'I didn't want to blend in with other people,' our 36-Year-Old was saying, who had now been holding forth to the room for at least ten minutes, barely halting the verbal torrent to draw breath. She clearly enjoyed having a captive audience, who, despite appreciating the harrowing parts of her story, had begun almost imperceptibly to move from an empathetic and supportive attitude, to thinking (in my case, anyway): You're not the only one in here who is having problems! Why do you think we're all sitting here waiting for treatment of our own? How do you know we aren't in an even worse position than you? She'd asked none of us for details.

The lady at whom she was now directing her verbal volleys was valiantly endeavouring to contribute a reply or two of her own, only to be ridden over roughshod by this juggernaut of chat... She did, now, slow down a fraction, but only to regather her strength before kicking on... I have to admit, perhaps uncharitably, that she was by now beginning to forfeit my earlier sympathy and admiration. However, I do accept that her outpourings were probably, and understandably, concealing her own concerns about the ultimate outcome of her treatment.

'I found I was the clown of the ward because I used to make people laugh...' One or two splutters could be heard as we tried to stifle our scepticism... 'I could see the pain in people's faces, so tried to make them feel better. I know it doesn't go away, but during those moments you're laughing you can at least feel a little better...'

She turned to the woman over whom she had verbally trampled for the past few minutes, before advising her: 'Tell your mum to keep on smiling – she has such a pretty smile.' There was a definite gasp-fest in the room.

A newbie lady now entered, and rescued us from what could have been an awkward moment or two, by asking whether she had to do any more than check in. We all hastened to reassure her, as 36-Your-Old started up again: 'LA3 is the worst – they really strap you down.' I interjected that I'd been there, and they hadn't strapped me down any more violently there than anywhere else I'd been, restraining myself from suggesting that they were trying to stop her flow of verbals by taking such action.

Still clearly unconvinced, the newbie went to tell the radiographers, who sat round the corner in their own little territory, that she had arrived. Once she sat down we were able to talk to each other and it transpired that, like me, she had a grandchild in New Zealand. It also transpired that her husband, like my wife, had found that he couldn't, because of sweaty fingers, convince one of the machines in a Los Angeles airport (en route to New Zealand) to authenticate his bona fides.

Again, like my wife, he had been taken off to an obscure part of the room and left to de-sweat sufficiently to try again... Clearly, this was not an enjoyable or even acceptable experience, neither for him nor my wife. But then, we agreed, neither of them was going to have to spend a good chunk of a morning listening to our 36-year-old fellow patient in full flow for what seemed like hours, were they?!

At my unexpected radiographer meeting I was talked through the entire radiotherapy process, which was obviously now well underway. He sounded confident that I wouldn't be required to have any extra treatment or procedures other than to continue the regular HRT injections for a two-year period. During this thorough check on my progress, a mention of the effects of Viagra came up. I'll resist any follow-up comment...

Back in the waiting room, my occasional companion, Very Tall Man, had arrived and was talking to Primary School Teacher – they were discussing some vintage TV programmes, none of which could ever be screened now for fear of mortally offending every viewer under the age of 60, and a considerable number of woke older ones. Amongst these classics of their type, were such hilarities as *Please Sir* (1968-72), *Till Death Us Do Part* (1965-75), *On the Buses* (1969-73) and the somewhat later *Mind Your Language* (1977-79). Probably best to pretend that *Love Thy Neighbour* (1972-76) didn't even exist!

However, there was a unanimous decision from all in the room that we are seriously offended by people – many of them permanently, er, not asleep – who claim to be offended at the drop of a hat, and who take to demanding 'safe spaces' to 'protect' themselves from hearing or seeing something which risks upsetting their poor, ultra-sensitive eyes and ears.

When I went to start drinking, I couldn't, as there were no cups there, so I legged it to reception and grabbed one, except that it was blue and a different shape from my usual model, the familiar white. I drank one blue cup before spotting an 'old-faithful' on the floor, so I checked the capacity of each, and there was significantly more volume available from the blue cup. I raised the matter with a passing medic who almost instantly produced a whole new supply of the white ones. I ended up drinking a combination of blue and whites, adding up probably to about five and a half whites.

It was by now 2.30 pm. I'd brought Melissa Etheridge along with me today – on CD, of course. As usual, the treatment room contained the laser machine with its adjustable bed. I walked in, once again not wearing a gown, despite being instructed to on day one. No one had ever objected. I removed my trainers and shed my jeans and my jumper; retained my T-shirt, polo shirt (well, it *is* winter outside) and underpants; then jumped up – or lifted myself, at least – on to the bed, and inserted my feet into what appeared to be the equivalent of sprint-race blocks a la Usain Bolt, leaned back and adjusted on to a headrest.

Then I was asked to confirm my birth date and the first line of my address, all designed of course, to ensure that the person on the slab is the one supposed to be there. My answers were matched against the information showing on a screen in the room, which also listed my details and treatment plan.

I'm now asked to put my arms and hands together on my chest. The radiographers shift me into place, warning me, 'Don't move, let us move you,' as they check references with each other as they go, moving me a fraction here, raising me a tad there. When they have agreed with each other that they're happy with their manoeuvres, they tell me they're off. But not before I've asked them to insert Melissa into the elderly CD player hiding in the corner of the room, looking outclassed and embarrassed alongside the state-of-the-art medical technology about to begin zapping me.

The radiographers now hasten out as the massively thick door slowly wheezes and closes in place, shutting firmly behind them, leaving me frozen in posture, petrified to move in case I'm suddenly and wrongly zapped in some orifice not supposed to receive behaviour of that nature. Initially it had seemed that the lights had to be dimmed, but this hadn't always been the case. From my inert, immobile position I looked up and could see about a dozen backlit panels on the ceiling depicting leafy tree branches. At this point I usually closed my eyes and listened to the music, trying to stop myself wriggling or twitching. You really learn just how difficult it is not to shift even a fraction, but trying to stay still outside of the treatment room proves *totally* impossible, whereas inside it, an additional level of self-defence kicks in to prevent even the slightest movement. My mind took over from the muscles and issued its own commands not to budge. Whether those in the control room were able to move the bed from there, I never found out – mainly as I didn't ask.

Maybe ten minutes later – I had asked one of the radiographers whether treatment times varied with each session and was told that they didn't – the buzzing, beeping, burping machine fell silent, the great doors began to creep open, and one or two of the radiographers marched in to lower the bed, loosen my bindings and let me jump off to pick up my belongings – including the CD – and head into the changing room.

Gradually, I felt my muscles unclenching as I relaxed and became less conscious of desperately trying to remain immobile. Exiting the treatment room and subsequently walking out past the waiting room which, like the water in a bath, had now reshaped itself to look as though you'd never occupied any part of it, I noticed the array of greetings cards, presumably from other grateful patients. I'd been wondering how best to express my thanks to these ministering angels for their cheerfulness, consideration and kindness, day in, day out. Bottles of wine, chocolates, personalised letters, telling them face to face?

Not more importantly, but certainly more urgently, I was now rushing into the gents to unload some of that H_2O before – now officially no longer a resident – I traipsed off to the bus stop at the end of this, my 6th week. Thirty sessions completed, nine remaining.

So, Melissa and I had completed treatment at shortly before 3 pm, and I was home an hour later when, turning into my road, a passing neighbour told me: 'I love your hat.' Home alone I pondered whether we waiting-room warriors were just comforting each other with our black humour... Was that our 'go-to' defence mechanism against facing the fact that probably some of us may not make it: may not be cured or may be only temporarily cured? Or that some of us may ultimately be receiving treatment of many kinds for the remainder of our life spans?

***

Saturday, of course a no-treatment day, became a difficult day. Having told Sheila that my review had suggested that things were proceeding to plan, I then had a weekend when I began to feel I might be losing all control over my bladder. I'd only had to get up twice overnight but then between breakfast and preparing to go and watch Wealdstone FC, I'd felt an urgency to urinate, and a stinging sensation when doing so, as well as beginning to experience a little, er, seepage, shall we delicately term the problem?

I relieved myself shortly before departing for the match at 2.30 pm, and as I'd hoped, the distraction of the game and talking to friends, helped me not to have to go again until I returned home at 5.30, and with the 'Stones' having lost the match 1-3 to Welling. I watched television in the evening, forcing myself to impose a three-hour ban on returning to the bathroom each time I needed to go.

In order to increase my chances of improving the gap between each dash to the toilet, I began stepping up my pelvic exercises, which take just a little repetition in order to become second nature, and can be done unobtrusively whilst seated. They did seem to have a positive effect and I do recommend that you get stuck into regular sessions should you ever find yourself in my position...

Things hadn't changed by Sunday morning. I was booked to go and see Wilko Johnson, formerly of successful group Dr Feelgood, playing at the Alban Arena – supported by one half of the most important duo in Squeeze, Glenn Tilbrook.

Johnson had famously been diagnosed with terminal pancreatic cancer but then stubbornly failed to die. Up against that my own condition struck me as trivial. I couldn't *not* go to the gig, so off we went, despite the somewhat depressingly wet weather which turned briefly to slushy snow as it fell.

We watched Tilbrook's good-humoured, enjoyable warm-up turn, complete with wry observations and self-deprecating stories. When he'd finished I knew I had to inspect the toilet facilities at the venue. Unusually, there was a far longer queue for men than for women. They couldn't all be PC patients, surely? Unless this was a special PC night for which my invitation had been lost in the post...

I began searching, increasingly urgently, for an alternative, even leaving the building and nipping into the nearby and still open branch of Ladbrokes, where I was unsmilingly informed between the staff (one man and one woman sitting punter-less behind the counter), that their facilities were 'out of order' – rather like the tone in which this information was delivered.

No problem, in the end: thanks to a secluded area of dustbins down a side road where I was able to enjoy an al fresco spilling of liquid. Needs must and all.

'You took your time,' said Mrs Sharpe.

'You don't want to know,' I told her.

Wilko's performance was enjoyable and lively, although he noticeably began to flag a little towards the end, clearly running out of gas. His rather knackered encore of Chuck Berry's 'Johnny B Goode' was strictly by numbers, but I empathised and certainly did not agree with those around me terming it: 'More like "Johnny B Bad".'

10

IN WHICH DOUBT KICKS IN

THE NEW week commenced as the old had ended – with a couple of morning evacuations of both types.

I had had no lunch before heading into Mount V where I discovered that I, in common with most of the regulars, had been diverted from LA10 to LA9, as 10 was being serviced. Walking down to the new location I spotted Pat, Mr Umpire and Sally:

'Standing room only in there,' warned Pat.

It was good to stand and catch up with their news – the Cheltenham Festival and Brexit featured on our agenda – but the apparently bigger revelation was that Sally had been suffering from 'skin burns' from her treatment, and yesterday had gone to A & E locally for some cream which, when she arrived here today, she was warned not to use directly before this afternoon's treatment. Sally was due to end her sessions at the end of the week.

They'd seen Barry, who was also finishing on Friday. 'Barry told the radiographers that as a result of his treatment, and the fact that his skin tans very quickly, he's acquired two strong black lines on his skin,' revealed Pat, who didn't seem to have seen the evidence.

'They told him they couldn't lighten them, so he said he wanted the same colour all over!'

By the time Sally emerged from the laser room we'd been joined by Very Tall Posh Man, who immediately took part in our Brexit deliberations, which resulted in a unanimous vote by five to nil, in favour of a No-Deal departure as quickly as possible, thus proving conclusively, depending on your point of view, that all male Brexiteers are prostate cancer patients, or that anyone who failed to vote Remain is certain to suffer from prostate cancer. Sally and co. departed, so Very Tall Posh Man and I wandered into the waiting room, where we were told they were running about an hour behind schedule.

Mondays so often appeared to be the busiest day. Suresh was presiding, with the blonde Rock Chick lady also present – I hoped she liked Wilko Johnson!

I kept to myself the fleeting thought that it must be natural for fellow cancer sufferers, who hear of someone who has had an amazing reprieve such as Wilko's, to feel secretly that their own survival odds will be lengthened. Possibly due to a combination of hearing about Sally, my weekend difficulties, not having had lunch, and now a potential lengthy delay, I did begin to have some darkish thoughts about the outcome of the remaining 14 treatments that I was yet to undergo. How would I feel by the end? Knowing that side effects could still kick in for perhaps a fortnight afterwards... Could it be a case of getting worse before it – if it – got better? And how would I cope?

A lady had gone in, but with just four of us remaining in the waiting room we were all staying quiet, though wondering why none of us had yet been asked to start drinking and who would be the first and last to receive such an instruction. Last week's newbie, Permanently-Flustered Margaret, had also arrived, but had been intercepted and diverted by Suresh to another location. Now another 'Very Tall Male' arrived this one notable for his penchant for always having a chat with the radiographers before bestowing his presence on us minions – and asked whether he had 'time to get some lunch' before going in.

It was just before 2.30 pm and Very Tall Male was told he should return no later than 3.30. However, with a 3.45 appointment and knowing that drinking doesn't start until there was about half an hour before you'd go in, he must have expected what he was told: 'You should be in at about 4.30.'

The patient I knew as John Buchan, despite having no idea of his progress, was sent off to LA3, before I was asked whether I could start drinking now and finish in five minutes. I made a valiant but unsuccessful attempt which left me feeling horribly swamped by 3.03 pm.

Yet another Tall Guy, this one from LA10 – and, yes, I am just the tiniest bit vertically challenged, so it is quite possible that you, dear reader, might not regard these daily inmates as particularly sky-scraping beings – came into the room. He was critical that Suresh had left a misspelled message on the door to LA10, explaining that it was out of order. Suresh hit back with: 'If I didn't put a message up, everyone would just sit in there waiting.' Which rather avoided the question of his poor spelling... My friend, the 'Here Every Day Nurse', walked past and called, 'Hello!' Suresh then suggested that LA10 might shortly be back in action.

My treatment passed uneventfully – except that when I stood up to go in, I complained that I couldn't find my glasses. 'On your nose,' observed another patient – with Rock Chick in charge, and Wilko Johnson sounding livelier on CD than he had at the end of his live show. However, the after-treatment situation was a little more eventful, as I was finding it difficult to dispense with some of the super-chilly water I'd taken on board, despite trying in three separate toilets.

I caught a 311 bus to Northwood Station where I shed some more liquid weight, but then discovered that thanks to signal failure the trains were badly disrupted, which sent me back into ablution mode before dashing off to catch an H11, which deposited me at my next stop just in time to miss my connecting H12. So I started walking instead and by the time I eventually made it home, I was just about done in (technical medical term, equating to the often used slang term 'knackered').

I was now two thirds of the way through my scheduled timetable.

***

Three bouts of increasingly damp diarrhoea on Tuesday morning, left me wondering whether I could make it to Mount V unscathed on this squally opening day of the Cheltenham Festival.

I thought I'd head in early, so for a 2.50 pm appointment I went to catch the 12.23 bus, but I'd left my bus pass behind and had to rush back, amazingly enough, returning in time for the 12.23 despite the windy and rainy weather.

It was still pouring with rain as I entered reception at Mount V, only for my mood to turn sunny as I spotted Ron who was just arriving for his 'Brachy treatment'. He'd been down to see the good folk of LA10, dispensing 'cakes and chocolates' to the radiotherapists. He was in a philosophical mood about what he was about to receive, and I said I'd give him a call the next week to hear all the gory details.

While we were talking, along came our Jehovah's Witness mate and I teased him that I was still waiting for the literature he'd promised me. He was heading towards LA3 and LA7, so I told him I was in LA10 and that he should nip along when he was finished.

In LA10 I found our loudly spoken 36-Year-Old patient, once again holding forth to her audience: 'I'm 36, but was only 35 when starting treatment,' she was telling two ladies who were then called in for a conversation with the radiographers. Undeterred, she just redirected her verbal volleys at the five of us left in the room, despite our less than enthusiastic expressions as she spoke at us. Now, I understand that, of course, she was probably endeavouring to hide her own nerves and insecurities, and she was entirely harmless, and quite humorous. But there are times when one should instinctively gauge the mood of an audience, and respond accordingly, even if that means just shutting up.

The odd 'Mm's and 'Really?'s were directed back at her with scant enthusiasm. However, in walked a lady pushing a gent in a wheelchair – the two immediately gained 36-Year-Old's undivided attention. There was already a half-hour delay – probably to enable staff to get stuck into Ron's goodies – which did little to halt 36-Year-Old's flow: 'Yesterday I was in 12, today I'm back home. The noise of the machine there was horrendous.' Most of the rest of us were obviously thinking, 'Yes, we know what you mean about horrendously loud noises.'

But she really had no volume control and now she was telling us about getting stuck in a lift with her sister: 'She said, "We're gonna die," so I told her in no uncertain terms: "Shut up!"' Would she take her own advice?

Er, no... 'Every time I go into a machine, I'm thinking, is it going to eat me alive? You have to laugh...' Finally, she began to wind down: 'This has been a good experience. This has opened my eyes to life. You have to fight.'

I tried to bury my head and ears in the copy of *Fortean Times* which I'd brought along – it specialises in stories of the unusual, bizarre and supernatural – only to discover that, unusually and bizarrely, I'd left it at home in my other 'hospital jacket'.

'When I go in they tell me to hold my breath for 17 seconds,' declared 36-Year-Old. No, dear reader, I am NOT making this up!

Rock Chick nurse appeared, and asked a patient to come in, apologising that the changing room was temporarily out of bounds, as it was being cleaned. 'But you can come straight in and not have to sit in here for longer with your legs crossed.'

'I thank my lucky stars I don't have to do the water drinking,' said the chap sitting next to me. I don't reply, but feel jealous of him.

Earlier that day my brother, Barry, had dropped me an email complaining about some after-effects from his recent hernia operation. I told him I reckoned that consultants deliberately downplay such potential effects beforehand, then tell you later they are what you should have expected and accepted. But you don't know that in advance, so think that the expected is actually the unexpected, causing some stress you might otherwise not have suffered.

I was jolted out of my 'escaping from 36-Year-Old' reverie by the arrival of Jehovah's Witness, clutching books and booklets, which he handed over to me, and asked whether I'd jot down his phone number, which I let him do for himself in the back of the notebook I brought along with me every day.

'Are you on WhatsApp?' Jehovah's Witness asked me.

'No idea,' I lied.

I'd probably see him again, as he had yet to finish his sessions.

A queue-jumper from LA7 arrived and was sent in ahead of the three of us left in the waiting room, and I was finally laid out on the slab at around 3.30 to the accompaniment of some Kate Bush, whose music invariably cheers me up and reminds me that Sheila and I saw her on her very first – and, for many years afterwards, her only – live appearance show, which was at the London Palladium, and was truly stunning.

I managed to make it home in time to watch the big race, the Champion Hurdle (albeit on ITV+1), from the Cheltenham Festival, in which I had placed my future financial wellbeing on the aforementioned Apple's Jade, currently my favourite horse. She wasn't my favourite horse after the race, in which she had run abysmally. Usually a front runner, she was not allowed to bowl along in front, and the writing was soon on the wall as, seemingly sulking at not getting her own way, she gradually drifted backwards.

If that wasn't bad enough, I consoled myself by eating a Cornish pasty, to dispose of which I later had to get up out of bed on three separate occasions.

***

The worst excesses of Pastygate had subsided by the time I had to drive Sheila to Waitrose the next morning. I was in a slightly more subdued mood than normal, so opted not to depart before the bookmaker's favourite time of day, 20 to 1, to board an H11, eventually arriving at Mount V an hour later, to find only one other patient already ensconced in LA10, who told me she had a 1.30 appointment.

More began to arrive, including a 30-something lady who said she was on her 31st radiotherapy treatment with a 'couple more to go' before she would then have some time off prior to commencing chemotherapy. Also arriving was an apprehensive-looking 60-plus lady, and a chap I vaguely recognised. The mood was somewhat downbeat and quiet.

A radiographer came in to give 1.30 Lady some anti-sickness medication to take before being treated. She wasn't overjoyed to receive this and protested that she had had radiotherapy before with no problem. 'Yes, but that was on a different area of your body,' she was told.

My notes tell me that at this point I thought to myself: 'Am I still seeing this whole experience just as material for a forthcoming book? If not, why I am writing it all down? Would anyone want to publish such a title?'

We all watched as 1.30 Lady swallowed her pills down – none of us, I think I'd be right in assuming, envied her at all at that moment. She was still miffed, and immediately screwed up the paper in which her pills had been contained.

Looking to lighten the mood, the newish lady sitting opposite declared: 'So, now we have a long wait – this is why we're called patients!'

The guy from yesterday added, 'I keep getting here early, because once when I did so, I was seen early.' Inwardly, I agreed with him. But then he offered the staggering insight that: 'There's a new thing which can tell you what your life expectancy is if you don't have treatment, and what it will be if you do.' Stunned silence all round for a while. I certainly didn't have any desire to know either of those options. Now the conversation turned to the ability of some, and not others, to solve cryptic crosswords, until a radiographer asked: 'Craig, would you be able to get changed, please?'

Guy From Yesterday, who had a 2 pm appointment, immediately leapt into action. At the same time, I realised I had forgotten to bring along the squash-infused water I'd prepared earlier, so I would have to face glugging neat hospital liquid. Oh well, I'd now done that 20-plus times, with another dozen to survive.

Guy From Yesterday confided: 'I'm having 20 treatments. I only have mild PC.' That's what I'd consoled myself by thinking – so how and why was I ending up getting 39, I kept wondering...?

For the first time throughout this entire process, I now genuinely began to think that maybe I'd been forgotten, or been dropped off the treatment list that day. The fellow ahead of me should have been done at 2.30 and here we were at 2.50 and he hadn't even started drinking. I could be sitting here until after 4 pm at this rate, I thought. Okay, so I had nothing else to do, but it was still a little irritating.

Sickness Pills woman went in before us. I think this was decided to make up for the mistake in not prompting her to take medication early enough to meet her scheduled appointment. I wasn't really enjoying that day's waiting room experience, I'm afraid.

When I was finally called – only about half an hour after my scheduled treatment time – the final disappointment of the day was that Santana was not turned up loudly enough on the CD machine, for which the radiographer later apologised, making me feel even worse by adding to his already burdensome workload.

Toilet stops: twice before departure, a couple more at Northwood Station and a reprise at Pinner Station got me home dry, by 5 pm.

Apart from the central heating playing up a bit, going off when it was supposed to be coming on, and vice versa, the evening passed without too much stress.

11

IN WHICH I WONDER WHETHER MATT'S FINISHED BY PC CRITICISM

ONE MIGHT have thought that the health secretary might be praised for getting himself checked out for future possible health risks. However, when Matt Hancock, who occupied that role in the government at the time, did just that and then revealed that he had discovered that he may have a higher-than-average chance of getting PC and that he planned to do something about it, he probably didn't expect to get a media and medical mauling.

The *i* website ran this story on 20 March 2019: 'Health Secretary Matt Hancock is at greater risk of prostate cancer after taking a genetic test that revealed his chances of getting the disease.' The article continued: 'In a speech at The Royal Society on Wednesday to celebrate the "100,000 Genomes Project", Mr Hancock is expected to say that a national debate to tackle some of the biggest ethical questions facing DNA testing is needed to allow patients to benefit from the revolutionary technology as soon as possible.'

Mr Hancock, said the website, was expected to say:

I recently underwent a predictive genomic test to better understand this technology and the ethical issues it presents. [The test] gives a sophisticated assessment of a person's likelihood to develop certain diseases based on their DNA.

I have to admit: I was pretty nervous about getting the results. The good news is I'm pretty healthy – below average for most of the 16 diseases [I was tested for]. I probably have my grandmother, who lived to 103, to thank for that.

But... I'm at higher risk of prostate cancer. My risk of prostate cancer by age 75 is almost 15 per cent. I was surprised, and concerned. Because I have no family history of prostate cancer. But I discussed what it meant with the doctor and when I realised that dying from prostate cancer is highly preventable if caught at an early stage and with regular checks, I felt hugely relieved.

Okay, that sounded fair enough to me. But not, it seemed, to *The Independent*, who declared that:

Matt Hancock has faced criticism from experts after claiming a controversial genetic test for cancer could have saved his life. He revealed details of the results, and said he was 'surprised and concerned' he was at an elevated risk of developing prostate cancer.

Writing in the *Times*, he said he was in the worst 10 per cent in the country for the disease, despite having no family history of it.

Professor David Curtis, from University College London's Genetics Institute, declared that Mr Hancock's response was 'a perfect example of someone "massively misinterpreting" such tests, which are often inaccurate.' The professor continued: 'As a health secretary, he displays a quite astonishing level of ignorance about the NHS. There is no such thing as a screening appointment for prostate cancer. We don't do them because they don't work, they're a waste of time and money, they cause unnecessary anxiety to patients.'

Professor Helen Stokes-Lampard, chair of the Royal College of GPs, reportedly said that 'Many things that will be picked up by genetic testing will be unimportant or of dubious value, and these could leave people unnecessarily confused and distressed. This will undoubtedly lead to an increased number of worried people wanting to visit their GP to discuss their borderline results, at a time when general practice is already struggling to cope with intense demand.'

Angela Culhane, the CEO of Prostate Cancer UK, also wagged a finger at Mr H in a letter published by the *Times* on 21 March 2019: 'we do not recommend investing privately in DNA tests as a first step for men concerned about their risk of prostate cancer.'

Looks to me, like some people can't do right for doing wrong. To me, anything encouraging men to be aware of the possibility of PC is to be encouraged.

Coincidentally, around the same time that the Hancock controversy was swirling around, a story in the *Times* on 18 March 2019 had an attention-grabbing headline: Prostate cancer is 'less deadly than thought'.

Chris Smyth, health editor, suggested in the story that 'doctors overestimate the deadliness of prostate cancer by more than 50 per cent, the creators of a test designed to give more accurate predictions say.' Well, one might think: 'They would say that, wouldn't they?'

But the article also suggested that doctors think treatments such as surgery or radiotherapy 'are five times as effective as they actually are'. The researchers, from Cambridge University, published a study for which they had asked 190 doctors and nurses to estimate patients' chances of survival in 12 case studies.

On average doctors estimated 15-year death rates at 24% compared with 15% calculated by the Predict model, which was derived from data on 10,000 British men... 'Most doctors don't have a clue,' Vincent Gnanapragasam, the consultant urologist who led the study, said... His study found that doctors estimated that an extra 25 lives per 100 patients would be saved by radical treatment, but the Predict model put the figure at 5 per 100.

A similar story in the *Daily Mail*, on 13 March 2019, reported that 'for a third of prostate cancer patients, or roughly 15,000 men in Britain [of the 47,000 men diagnosed], the chance of dying is so low that choosing to have surgery or radiotherapy will provide little benefit.'

Two thirds of NHS hospitals were reportedly now using MRI scans to diagnose PC, reported the *Times* on 17 June 2018. This followed a trial the previous year which had shown that it was the most accurate method currently available.

12

IN WHICH THE WEEK ENDS POSITIVELY

THE NEXT morning, following the now-regulation three bowel evacuations – one normal, two gushers; since you ask – I decided not to rush to Mount V in the hope of an early exit, such as had proved somewhat illusory of late.

I arrived at 1.40 pm to find John Buchan already in earnest conversation with a lady, discussing the 'reinvention of Boris Johnson'. John had been in LA12 yesterday, and anticipated the same venue today, only to receive a call 'at 6 am this morning, asking me whether I would like to come at 1.20 or 4 pm today. I chose 1.20 and they told me to come here to LA10... but now it's already 1.45.'

He was, though, called shortly after that, and asked whether he had 'emptied'. 'Yes, half an hour ago,' he confirmed.

'Would you mind emptying again, just for us?' came the response. So off he bustled.

I later heard Mr Buchan requesting 'that thing I can get to show in shops, etc, if I'm out and get taken short.' I was surprised that he hadn't received one at his introductory pre-treatment meeting.

The chap due to go in one ahead of me was asked to start drinking well before 2 pm. We looked at each other, wordlessly wondering whether this might mean we'd both get in early for a change. He returned after completing his quaff, but no one appeared to check his finishing time as they usually did. He told me that his review was due today but that, as ever, he'd been given no specific time. That would spoil the effect of going in early if he then had to sit around afterwards, awaiting his review.

I was sent out for drinking at 2.31 and was met by Jolly Woman at the fountain – a good-humoured lady who inevitably drank much faster than me. If you recall, she had introduced herself initially by guffawing at my drinking pace and calling me firstly a 'wuss' and then a 'wimp'.

'How many sessions?' she quizzed.

'39.'

'My God – you'll be glowing!' she joked. Well, I HOPED she was joking. She then told me she'd just seen a young girl with a baby, waiting for treatment. 'I feel sorry for them at that age,' she added, not making it clear whether she meant she felt sorry for the baby or for the young girl, or both of them. We agreed that dealing with a situation like this was somewhat easier for us, given that we acknowledged we had already had a substantial life – not that we actively wished it to be shortened though – and were probably better equipped to deal with what life now decided to throw our way at this stage. We're half expecting it, anyway, if we are honest.

'I think a positive mindset is important – and to be grateful that at least there is treatment offered to us.'[1]

I chucked in some thoughts: that it was important to accept early on that your dignity no longer mattered, and that it was pointless to get upset at the various inevitable embarrassing or invasive treatments which were all for your own ultimate benefit. She looked closely at me: 'At least you haven't lost your hair.'

'... yet.' I said – conscious that I had no idea whether it could be a casualty of the radiotherapy somewhere along the line.

Today I was conversing with David (2.30 appointment) and Asian Man (2.45). Asian Man told us he'd just been reading a news story asserting that a system was about to be introduced, enabling patients to be assessed and told what their life expectancy might be, if (a) they accepted treatment or (b) declined the same.

'I don't want to know,' he averred. David and I both agreed.

A bigger shock was to hear from David that he had already had his prostate removed, yet he was now back on radiotherapy, as his

---

1. I should probably remind readers at this point, that I was writing this part of the book at the time – November 2020 – when many non-covid conditions were suffering delayed or cancelled treatments.

PSA had begun to rise at his regular check-ups, thus indicating that they hadn't managed to take it all out. He seemed philosophical about this. I wasn't sure whether I would feel the same in his place.

With a little help from The Who's Greatest Hits, today's treatment was comparatively straightforward.

***

It surprised me each day just how few people arrived at Mount V via omnibus transport – I don't think I have ever personally disembarked with more than four other patients or staff, and saw very few arriving on the other routes which terminated there – yet nearly every day someone complains to me about the hassle of getting into the car park. Of course, the distances involved for some make bus travel a non-starter.

Still, this day, Friday, 15 March, the final day of my 6th week, I was convinced a fellow traveller, clad in thick jerkin and woolly hat, and looking pretty much at death's door, was a definite fellow-patient.

But no, two stops from Mount V he leapt from his seat and jumped off, leaving just two of us to arrive at the hospital.

It was about 1.45 when I (2.45 appointment) and David (2.30) were asked to drink.

I'd had my now customary ordinary/gusher/mini-gusher bowel evacuation session that morning, which certainly would have made life and travel awkward had I still been on morning sessions, which was possibly something taken into account when patients were being given treatment times. A lady using crutches returned to the waiting room following her session – which was focused on her leg. 'It really hurts, because of the position I have to keep my leg in.'

'Oh well,' I replied, 'at least you have the consolation of knowing it is making the leg better.'

'No – that's the other one, this one just has to be kept out of the firing line!'

I told her about bringing my own CDs along to listen to – Cat

Stevens, today – and she revealed a love of classical music, then told me of a friend, whose husband had come in for his treatment and kept the rest of the waiting room entertained each day whilst waiting for his turn:

'So much so, that one man who was just about to finish his treatment asked whether he could return each day so as not to miss the regular entertainment he was enjoying so much.'

'Wow, sounds like that chap was a bit of a character.' I responded.

'Yes... it was Roy Castle.'

Roy Castle, a very popular entertainer, actor, musician and presenter, died of lung cancer in September 1994. In late 1991 Professor Ray Donnelly had carried out the first removal of a lung cancer by keyhole surgery which brought international publicity.

Professor Donnelly recalled how Roy came to be involved with what became the Roy Castle Lung Cancer Foundation: 'In 1993 I put together my ideas for an international research facility in Liverpool and it was then that we went to Roy Castle and asked for his help. His response was magnificent and, although he was dying, we arranged a "Tour of Hope" by special train around the UK which raised over £1m in three days during July 1994.'

The Roy Castle Lung Cancer Foundation website continued:

At each of the towns and cities where the train stopped, Roy and his wife Fiona would emerge to entertain thousands of people who turned out to hail his talent and bravery, and offer contributions to our cause. As Professor Donnelly adds: 'His contribution to our development cannot be exaggerated. He was with us for only eight months but in that time, he captured the hearts of the nation. He is still very fondly remembered. After Roy died... I proposed to the trustees that we should put his name on to the charity and so we became the Roy Castle Lung Cancer Foundation.'

As I was finishing the day's activities, and whilst listening to Cat Stevens' song 'I Love My Dog' – I have, by the way, no affection for canines whatsoever, having been bitten by members of the species on four different occasions whilst out running, although I have been known to show love for racing greyhounds if and when they win races for which I have backed them – I asked the radiographer whether I now qualified for a special badge, having completed my 30th session.

He looked at me: 'As we say in my culture, the elephant has passed, just the tail remains to pass.' Is he suggesting I bear some resemblance to a pachyderm, I wondered inside my head, before responding: 'And as we say in my culture, do you think you could please turn the music up a bit louder in future?'

I then explained all about Cat Stevens' odd and lengthy career break and recent return to more mainstream activities – although I'm not anticipating anything to rival 'Matthew and Son' or 'Lady D'Arbanville'.

Over the weekend I worked hard to remain regular. I went immediately before heading off to Kenilworth Road for the week's torture afternoon, and managed to go once at the ground during the disappointing 2-2 draw with Gillingham.

Overnight I had to get up twice, and I was a little apprehensive about going to lunch with a very good friend's sister and her fellow – a 40-minute drive away. I went before leaving, on arrival, after our pub lunch and as soon as we walked back through the door at home.

All in all, though, a positive week's work.

13

IN WHICH I FEEL CORNERED

TWO PEARLS of wisdom got the week underway. Both received from Young-To-Middle-Aged Guy – someone I hadn't seen previously – as I walked into the familiar LA10 waiting room to hear the tail end of someone's complaint about the length of time they'd been waiting. 'It's not long when you consider how long life is,' responded Young-To-Middle-Aged-Guy.

Then a discussion of the time allowed between urinations began, with Young-To-Middle-Aged-Guy revealing that – 'I hold it until five or six miles from home, then stop the car and go,' – but without revealing where and how the 'go' part was happening.

The previous week had seen my own waterworks going somewhat haywire during the day, albeit not so much overnight – I was only up once this last night. I'd been struggling to maintain a couple of hours' gap between each daytime urination, not helped by feeling that each episode failed to leave me feeling completely empty. Perhaps this was linked to a lack of hydration, I thought, as I'd been told to try to be empty on arrival at Mount V so that I'd have the right amount in me for the upcoming session.

Bowel-wise, this day produced a typical ordinary/semi-gush/ gusher trio. Weather-wise, I survived a couple of light showers on the trip over, but it was a little warmer than of late.

I was scheduled for 2.55 pm and had brought a particular favourite for musical consumption: the Hollies' *Evolution* LP. It's quite a modern record – in my terms, anyway – from 1967. No time ago at all, really!

I sat quietly, pondering how much psychology or power of thought was involved in my current urination variables. It certainly seemed easier to cope when I was in a social situation which might embarrass me if I needed to go urgently. Once that aspect was absent, the urge invariably became more intense.

With nine treatments still remaining – almost another third on top of what I'd already done – I didn't want to start kidding myself I'd almost made it through.

Suddenly I heard: 'I feel sorry for you girls when you have to have an anagram...' (Mammogram, I presume the 'Jack the Lad'-looking speaker, who was addressing a lady I didn't know, meant...) 'It must feel like being put in a Breville.' He didn't elaborate on which

Breville product he meant – a kettle? Toaster? Blender? Sandwich maker? We're all baffled that he briefly brought up Breville.

At this point the radiographer enters and asks the man whether he wants to wait and start his drinking process again, or hold the water in for an extra 10 to 15 minutes before going in. Jack opts to wait and tells us all that he is going to have his alignment tattoos turned into a tattoo of the name 'Mount Vernon'. Somehow, we don't disbelieve him.

But the conversation now becomes a little more normal, as one of our number declares that 'two coffees, tea and a cake came to twenty quid'. He'd been to the nearby Ye Olde Greene Man pub and felt he'd been overcharged. Most of us agreed with him. Unless, of course, he'd eaten the whole cake and not just a slice...

Jack commented, 'I'd have just turned round and said I'm off. But then I don't drink, so have no idea of pub prices.' We were very surprised.

It was my turn. An uneventful one except for the CD player making my Hollies album jump all over the place, which was irritating. Perhaps I'll suggest they trade it in for a Breville.

***

The forecasters were predicting 'comparatively warm weather' for Wednesday, 20 March. Spring at long last, perhaps?

But, no, it was blooming chilly en route, although I warmed up when I had returned to LA10, to be greeted with a comedy moment, as a lady who was trying to open her bottle of drink prompted a bald gentleman to offer his help. He leaned across and promptly spilled his own cup of water all over himself.

A young lady leapt into action and fetched paper towels. Philosophically, the bald gentleman told us: 'No good deed goes unpunished.' A comment which we all lapsed into comparative silence to consider.

Another of the ladies in the room, having clearly considered something different, looked at me and said accusingly, but accurately: 'You always sit in the corner, don't you?'

As I was sitting in the corner my options were few, so I confessed to this terrible sin, omitting that it made it easier for me to watch, hear and record what they were all up to. Hopefully, she thought it was so that fewer people would notice how scruffy I was by now, having vowed to have neither hair cut nor shave until I'd completed my treatment. Something to do with new beginnings, I supposed...

My hale and hearty lady friend, Jolly Woman, who poured scorn on my drinking technique – 'Just swallow the stuff as quickly as possible, man!' – each time she saw me struggling with the process, was in the same waiting room as me today, along with her husband, when a grimly humorous Scottish nurse came in to deal with a problem Jolly Woman was having with her foot, on which the skin apparently frequently splits. The nurse handed over tablets, and rubbed in cream, explaining how she had been struggling to take time off that was due to her, because of patient demand. She was trying – and blatantly failing – to convince us that she only did her job under protest. She was clearly addicted to helping others and was typical of the vast majority of people I'd come across during my time here.

On Thursday, I was finally rumbled, when Roy Castle Lady asked me what I was writing in my notebook... then followed up by asking whether I'd ever had anything published. I told her I'd always earned a living from writing – from reporter, to press officer, to author – and I wrote things down as and when they struck me as potential material. My sieve-like memory guarantees I otherwise won't be able to recall what it is I know I should remember, but seem to have forgotten just as I start to tell someone.

I tell her about my latest book, a biography of the amazingly wealthy and eccentric racehorse owner, Dorothy Paget, who lived a topsy-turvy life, frequently staying up all night, eating huge meals after midnight then sleeping during the day. She lived in a large house staffed round the clock by a posse of female staff. Widely believed to be childless, largely because of her sexual proclivities, I discovered a man living not far away from Mount V, who claimed to be her son.

By the time I was finished and away, having listened to some satisfyingly three-chord Status Quo rocking, I found myself in the midst of mayhem, as a mob of manic bus-boarding schoolkids trampled all opposition underfoot. As usual, I managed to squeeze into a corner, keep quiet, keep my head down, and arrived home at 4.30 pm.

***

It was the last day of my penultimate week of daily treatment. In one way these had been the worst seven or eight weeks of my life in terms of stress and strain. But also, the most enlightening and eye-opening, in terms of realising how many people there are stoically suffering, day in, day out, but keeping their problems to themselves. In the process, they inspire others in the same boat to feel more confident that they can not only cope but, with help, look forward to some kind of recovery and return to normality, albeit probably a new kind of normal.

After our recent conversations, I handed over a copy of my Dorothy Paget biography to Roy Castle Lady. She had told me that she had googled both Dorothy and me, so I thought she would enjoy reading the book.

She'd found someone with almost the same name as me who also writes books – although it wasn't the former Everton and Scotland footballer, whose name sounds the same as mine but is spelled differently. This has resulted in one or two occasions during our overlapping careers, as footballer and bookie-press officer-cum-public relations guru, when we each have been mistaken for the other and invited to be interviewed, only realising too late that we're being asked about the other's area of expertise!

No, she had come across a different, but similarly named writer. 'Did you ever consider changing your name?' she wondered.

'No, I suspect I've had the name longer than him, so if either of us should change, it should be him.'

'Before you actually told me your name, I'd given you one I considered appropriate – Indiana Jones – because of the hat, I think.'

'I'll accept that...' It appeared that other regular patients gave their fellows appropriate names, then.

Fellow waiting-room resident Dave told us he was into ancestry and he had been trying to track down a relative who seemed just to have vanished without trace, possibly in Australia. The subject of relatives enlivened Roy Castle Lady, who now informed us that although her direct family was 'dull', she was related to someone who had a horse race named in his honour in Ireland. She couldn't remember his surname, but he was called Denny, and had something to do with rock group Procol Harum...

This instantly resulted in a spark of recognition in the depths of what passes for my mind: 'Denny Cordell,' I suggested. I knew full well he was a record producer and had worked with many bands, including the 'Whiter Shade of Pale' boys.

'Yes, that's it!' said Roy Castle Lady. 'But I don't think Cordell was his real name. My name is Lavarack.'

It didn't take me long to check that Denny Cordell's full name was, indeed, Denny Cordell-Lavarack. Not only that, but after retiring from producing rock records he had become a horse racing trainer. Sadly, born in 1943, he had died in 1995.

To commemorate him, a horse race called the Denny Cordell-Lavarack Fillies Stakes was introduced at Gowran Park racecourse in 1996. It was created by his family and friends, who sponsored the race over one mile, one furlong and 100 yards. Amazing what you can learn in a radiotherapy waiting room!

David departed the building just after 3 pm. I'd finished drinking nine minutes earlier, vowing that when this 39-session nightmare was over, I would not voluntarily drink more than one glass of water at a time unless it was enforced at the point of a gun.

Today my drinking matter had been laced with some kind of

orange and peach concoction, which at least slightly eased the cold water 'taste'. Forget the incontinence and diarrhoea, *this*, the excessive H_2O, is the low point of the whole treatment ordeal – genuinely feeling when you are finished, with swollen stomach, as though you were pregnant (I imagine!).

And, what's worse, it was becoming an increasingly close-run thing not to leak on the laser table. I had, though, thus far managed to avoid disgracing myself in such a manner. I was maintaining that proud record this afternoon, although it was all the more difficult than usual to remain steadfastly still while Roxy Music wailed away at a proper kind of volume as the machine seemed to dance in time to 'Virginia Plain'.

But all of a sudden, I began to feel as though I needed to pass wind and at almost the same time, the heavy doors began to open again, yet I knew I was nowhere near the end of my session...

The radiographer walked in and greeted me with a phrase I'd never knowingly heard directed at me before: 'You have excess gas in the relevant area targeted by the laser, which is obscuring the image. Do you feel you could pass it – preferably also without passing any water? Otherwise we'll have to abandon this attempt and start the whole process again later on...'

This was basically a no-brainer. I couldn't possibly face the water ordeal twice in one day, so I said I'd give it a go.

Pulling on the odd piece or two of clothing, I was dispatched into the gents where I managed to dispel some of the offending clouds of gas, at the cost of considerable personal dignity, yet with minimal water wastage, before sneaking back into the laser room, as though nothing had really happened, resuming the required position and recommencing the session, to the strains of 'Do the Strand.'

Once completed the technicians declared that the session was deemed to have gone as planned, much to my, er, relief. Which was even greater some while later, when, having evacuated rather more than just gas from the offending region, I was able to regard the situation as stable enough to attempt the journey home, thus completing my penultimate week's treatment in unexpected style.

During the weekend I seemed to be feeling permanently as though I needed to pass urine. When I also discovered that I had managed to crack a tooth, my misery was complete.

I began to worry about the psychological side of irregular urinations. I was by now desperately hoping that all of this would improve gradually once I had finally finished my 39th session on the Thursday. But I wasn't feeling optimistic that I would be back to normal by the time – just a couple of weeks away – that Sheila and I were due to be flying out to San Francisco, a venue she had been desperate to visit for many years.

My mood was not enhanced either by reading a story in no less a respected organ than the *Times*, suggesting that 'precautionary radiotherapy' as it was called in the article, such as I and my fellow patients had been having, was pointless.

So, yes, one way or another, I was definitely feeling well and truly pissed off.

14

IN WHICH THE END IS NEAR

TRAGEDY SUDDENLY crashed in to remind me that, stressed though I may have been, there were others far worse off, as buses in and out of part of my route to Mount V were diverted and rerouted. This was following the owner of a local newsagent's being murdered during a botched robbery over the weekend.

On this day I had invited Sylvia, or Roy Castle Lady, whose husband, it transpired, used to own or run – or both! – The Tenby pub in Jersey (a regular holiday haunt of mine), and was born and buried there, to come and join my wife and I at our booked table at the Jersey Derby race meeting scheduled for 21 June.

Sylvia had never been to the races before, she said, but she was enjoying the Dorothy Paget book I'd given her, and was complimentary about the research which had gone into it.

I went in about half an hour after my scheduled time today. As ever I was routinely asked how I was, knowing full well, that giving any sort of detail would merely produce polite indifference.

At last, one of my musical choices sparked a little recognition – the 20-something radiographer looked surprised, and told me, 'Oh, I think I recognise that one,' as my CD choice of the day began with The Kinks' 'You Really Got Me'. Proof though that I am officially old/ancient/past it, arrived today via my disgust at the young mother on the bus home who allowed her younger son – 12-years-old, perhaps – to lay over two seats with his dirty trainers on them, while she just stared at her phone during the entire trip.

I felt absolutely exhausted during the evening, only managing to give a very good episode of one of my favourite programmes, *Alan Partridge*, minimum concentration.

I retired to bed at 10.30, thinking that the cumulative effect of the last seven weeks had really kicked in now, and worrying about how long it might take to return to anything like normal, or whether I actually would ever do so...

***

With the 3-2-1 countdown underway, I was sent out on loan from LA10 to 9. What price loyalty? I thought. After all, LA10 wasn't closed. Oh, well, off I went, wondering whether I might bump into Spurs-Fan David on his final day, or Sylvia, for more Jersey chat.

My waterworks were all over the place this day – one minute having to make a desperate dash, then feeling I wouldn't need to go for the rest of the day. I remained convinced that psychological factors were playing a significant part in this. I'd also had a disturbed night, with three trips downstairs – on one of them dropping my torch and waking up the household.

A notification from Facebook had alerted me to a slightly older cousin, Vivienne, who now lived in Canada, telling me that she's having to give up the line-dancing class she ran – and she'd won awards for it – because of an unspecified medical issue.

Viv has two sisters: Jill and Janice. The three of them lived with my eccentric uncle Charlie and lovely aunty Bet, in Shoeburyness near Southend, and we used to visit for idyllic, traditional 1950s, Enid Blyton-style summer holidays when we were very young.

As I arrived at the door of LA9, an elderly gent with a walking stick came in to tell his wife he was ready to depart. On the way out he looked at the five of us still sitting in the waiting room, raised his stick and said, 'Good luck!' in what struck me as an echo of the old prisoner-of-war movies with the never-say-die spirit of the inmates being somehow called upon in a hospital setting.

Sheila had said to me that morning, as we drank our tea (for me, decaffeinated = horrible) and coffee (for her, strong, no sugar = lovely): 'Just a 3-2-1 to go now.' She was just giving me a boost, but I still thought to myself, and it was, of course, partly my own fault: I'm not sure she quite knows how gruelling this has been. I only hoped it would all have been worthwhile in the end.

With the end in sight (interpret that phrase how you wish) I'd booked an appointment with my GP for 11 April to check whether he'd be happy for me to go to San Francisco with Sheila a couple of weeks later.

Number 9 was very quiet, no chatting happening. Perhaps I should go looking for Spurs-Fan Dave if he doesn't show up, I was thinking, as I had some spare time before my appointment.

I'd decided to do today's water drinking 'neat' – adding squash had merely succeeded in making me feel sick on the majority of occasions, and I also wondered whether it aggravates the bladder. Let's hope, I thought, I can force down the 18 remaining cups without any added ingredients.

Back in the waiting room, I literally fell asleep for a few minutes. When I awoke there were still none of my LA10 friends to be seen, although at 2.50 pm our Asian Gentleman came in, giving me a wave as he walked in, clearly also pleased to see a familiar face. It is surprising what a morale boost that can give. A man who'd been sucking on fruit sweets since he had arrived, without offering them around, went in before me, but eventually I was called in and with Eddy Grant's assistance, completed my 37th session.

As I departed to catch my bus on the penultimate-treatment morning, Sheila smiled, called me 'darling' and gave me a kiss. You may have gleaned from my ramblings that I am not often outwardly affectionate, but this gesture did touch me. I wondered how she had been affected by the whole situation, and realised that she clearly understood how I'd been feeling, even if I had not quite realised the effect on her. Mea culpa.

I met long-term waiting-room companion John Buchan as I arrived at Mount V: 'One more to go!' he greeted me.

'Me, too – well, when I've done today's one,' I responded.

I nipped into the gents before checking in, then discovered I was staying in LA9 for today, with a scheduled time of 2.40 pm. As I walked into the otherwise empty waiting room, I was informed by a radiotherapist: 'There's no one else here, so can you start drinking, please?'

I'd finished drinking at 1.44 and returned to sit in the waiting room where I was joined by a newbie, Anthony. We soon struck up a conversation about hospital A & Es, followed by pop groups and a discussion of the significance of Scott Walker's recently announced death.

I pointed out to Anthony that none of the three Walker Brothers were related to either of the others, but kept to myself the painful memory of a teenage girlfriend dumping me to camp at Heathrow Airport, waiting for Scott Walker to fly in, out, or off, taking her with him. Then we veered off to how well, or otherwise, PC was diagnosed. Anthony had had blood tests, but without a PSA test included, so it was essentially only detected by accident. It was his second day, but he'd been here before some 40 years ago: 'It looked exactly the same then.' Which made me think back to my own only previous experience of Mount V some 40-plus years earlier, when my 27-year-old good friend, Alan, had been treated here for the cancer which killed him.

I only got one track played from *Revolver* by The Beatles, while I was being treated, as the machine took it on itself to start with the final track and then assumed it had fulfilled its purpose. The radiographer apologised that the session had taken longer than usual: 'We were doing your weekly scan, which takes a bit longer, but it was all fine. Fab.' Well, that's good news. I hoped.

I headed home with mixed feelings. I'd obviously become a little institutionalised, as I definitely felt I would miss the routine when it was over. Not only for the regulars I'd met, but because it took away the responsibility for having to chart your own day when you woke up and after many years of having to do that in my work, I appreciated just going with the flow as instructed.

I was clearly a little discombobulated the next morning, as it was only once I'd arrived at Mount V, having taken three wee breaks en route, that I realised I had forgotten to bring my prized man-bag – the one purchased on a visit to New Zealand – in which I'd carefully stashed today's intended final CD by The Pretty Things. Not only that, but it contained my check-in card, so I had to queue at reception like a newbie on my last day – how demeaning for me, a grizzled veteran!

Naturally, the world's most disorganised and untidy female was ahead of me in the queue, endeavouring to arrange four appointments, tests and referrals. We were together with one sweet, elderly and bald lady, who took just 30 seconds to make her query and receive an answer.

'Can I help you?' asked a smiling receptionist.

'Today, 28 March, is the 39th of my 39 scheduled appointments.

I've remembered to bring my check-in card for all the others, but not today...'

'Don't worry. No pressure. What's your DOB? ...Ah, yes... you're in LA10.'

Back home for the final session, then. Good. Off I toddled, to find the chap I'd met over the past day or so waiting to be called, having done his drinking. When he went in, I checked they knew I'd arrived. A minute or two later, Suresh asked me to start drinking.

At bloody last – just six horrible plastic cups of freezingly foul water to force down, having already managed to quaff 228 of the bastard things. Somehow, hating and heaving all the way, I drove the liquid down and returned to await my last lie down on the laser merry go round, ironically finishing as I'd begun, with innocuous, inappropriate music playing around me.

After I'd finished, I gave the charming young lady, who'd been so good with my music over the weeks, the card and chocolates I'd brought along with which to say some small thank you to all of those who were, of course, 'Only doing their jobs'.

They asked me to wait, before handing over some final information, together with a book of bleeding obvious tips for after you're done with the sessions, and a sheet of similar stuff. They told me when my telephone review would take place, and that was it. Off you go. Cheerio. Next, please.

But how else could it be? To them a job, to us, potentially a life-saving or life-extending adventure.

I went for a wee, reluctant to depart, looking for an excuse not to. I decided to have another wee in a gents close to reception, and was able to say goodbye to Sylvia on the way – reminding her to come and see me in Jersey. Reader, she didn't.

Then I was walking to the bus stop. Soon, I was home. At a loose end. Wondering how I would be filling my days going forward. How I'd cope without the informal, protective group I'd managed to form around me, at the same time, thinking how I'd no longer be a part of other patients' own protective groups. We were united by our individual roles in the daily random gatherings, as part of which we didn't need to explain why we were there, or what we were hoping to recover from, because we were all in the same, effectively anonymous, cancer commune.

***

A while down the line in August 2020, I read an interesting letter, sent to the *i*, which certainly resonated with me. It was written by Tony Mayston of Buckinghamshire, who had been diagnosed with PC in 2015 and received 'very good treatment' at Churchill Hospital in Oxford, and was now in remission. Wrote Tony: 'When I was diagnosed I consulted a friend who had been through it two years before and he proved to be most comforting and helpful. I had 37 days of treatment and as the scheduling meant it was the same men at the same time, we developed a sort of social club.'

Exactly. My thoughts precisely. That final day subsequently stayed prominently in my mind. The end of a significant, potentially life-saving or life-changing period. But for those looking after me whilst I lived it, how, I wondered, did they regard me and their other patients? Were we distinct, individual human beings, or just the tools of their trade – here this week or month, gone but quickly replaced afterwards, never to be thought of again?

Some while later I was able to contact one of them individually to ask for her thoughts on the job she does and how it affects her and her patients. I will keep her name out of what follows, although she didn't ask me to. This is what she told me:

I'm glad to hear your experience at Mount Vernon was good. No, being forced to listen to the Spice Girls definitely isn't everyone's cup of tea!

I think it does help patients being able to listen to their own music, and just passes the time a bit quicker. They can focus on that, rather than listening to the radiographers doing all their measurements.

I first started working at Mount Vernon Hospital eight years ago, working in a different department as an assistant. I was 18 and it was my first job that I had really enjoyed after doing several office jobs, and working in a pub.

I just really enjoyed working with the patients, and liked the feel Mount Vernon had as everyone was so nice to work with.

Three years ago I saw a job advertised in radiotherapy to progress as an assistant practitioner. It sounded like a role I'd really enjoy, and I thought it would be nice to have a change in a new department but also still be at Mount Vernon. I've now learnt so much about radiotherapy, and have found it all very interesting and really enjoy my job as I am not just based in one place, and can be all over the hospital on different treatment machines etc.

Due to Covid, we now don't have people waiting in the waiting rooms, we have a dedicated check-in phone, so this means patients call us to check in, which we then do on our system.

They wait in their car until we are ready for them to come in for their treatment.

For patients on transport, because there are not too many of them, they can continue to wait in the rooms.

I have always had a good experience with patients. Everyone is usually so positive and grateful. Sometimes it can be hard seeing patients upset. This is quite rare, surprisingly, but just having someone there to listen to can make a huge difference, and having a familiar face to see each day when they come for treatment can help a lot.

Meeting so many different people, and seeing some of them for a few months you really get to know them and they have interesting stories from their past. Some of the older patients who live alone and are quite lonely actually say they feel quite sad when treatment is over. We can get them into different services when they finish treatment, such as "befriending groups" and other things in the community.

If we did ever have to move from the current site, I would consider it and I'd also see what else was going on around me, and take it from there.

I'd begun to hear rumours that there were plans afoot to move the unit elsewhere.

***

In the evening after my final session had been completed, I rang Ron from St Albans, to see how his 'brachy' treatment had gone. 'I laughed my way through it,' he said, before giving me some appropriately gory detail. And I believed him. 'We've both come through positively,' he added.

I said I'd be over to meet up with him soon. And here, in his own words is what he told me about his 'brachy' experience and the lead-up to it...

15

IN WHICH WE HEAR RON'S STORY IN HIS OWN WORDS

By Ron Arnold

THINKING BACK, I probably should have realised that something was not quite right.

Five years ago, I noticed that my waterworks were not quite functioning as they should. Pee-breaks were getting more frequent, the flow weaker.

Being a bloke of a certain age – early 70s – I ignored the signs until, in June 2018 I attended the motorbike 'Autojumble' at Kempton Park Racecourse, where I bought a few bits for my old bike, had a cheeseburger with onions and a can of Diet Coke.

Back home by about 3 pm, I felt a slight pain in the area of my left kidney at about 4.30. By 6 pm the pain had intensified, until

I was feeling nauseous. Before long I was 'talking to the big white telephone' in the bathroom, where I had on numerous previous occasions conversed with the plumbing, but nothing compared with this occasion. Stomach emptied, I drank loads of water, had an early night, and blamed the 'dodgy' cheeseburger.

Four weeks later, a similar incident. Worse pain. No cheeseburger involved. The vomiting was worse. It lasted longer.

Two weeks later, a third episode. But the pain was now excruciating. After consulting with the plumbing again I just went and lay on the bed. The pain would not go away. I remember sitting on the edge of the bed, literally crying with pain.

In desperation, I rubbed Voltarol into the area between the bottom of my ribcage and the top of my pelvis. I pushed my fingers into the gap – suddenly, as if someone had flicked a switch, the pain was gone.

My wife had gone across the road to see our neighbour, Emma, a paramedic. Emma came in and proceeded to poke, prod, tap and listen to the affected area. She diagnosed trapped wind, and suggested it would be a good idea to see my GP.

The appointment took place in the first week of August 2018. Dr Cooper asked me loads of questions, before she suggested to me that I should have an 'internal probe'. It was at this point I realised that she suspected something a little more significant than trapped wind. Having donned plastic gloves and greased the fingers thereof, Dr Cooper completed the internal probe, and mentioned that my prostate was 'enlarged and misshapen'.

An ultrasound scan was booked, to be carried out at the Maltings surgery in St Albans. Arriving at the consulting room I was told to lay on a bed, pull my T-shirt up and push the top of my jeans down.

I then had 'jelly' spread on my, er, belly, while a scanner was rubbed around. 'You have a slightly fatty liver,' Dr Cooper said. I resisted the temptation to suggest: 'Okay, all we need now is a bit of bacon, tomatoes and kidneys for a mixed grill.'

A week later I was back at Dr Cooper's for my ultrasound result. She reiterated the fatty liver warning, adding that I should lose some weight and that perhaps my recent episodes of pain and nausea might be due to a kidney stone. The doctor made me an appointment for a PSA blood test, and another with a urologist at the City Hospital, which was confirmed for 17 September 2018 at 1.30 pm, together with instructions to bring a bottle of water to ensure a half-full bladder.

Jan and I arrived on time and I was escorted to a special toilet, where I was told to pee in what looked like a bucket with a trapdoor in the bottom, with gauges and wires around it. The nurse motioned to a ply panel in the wall, and said she would go into the room on the other side, and when she tapped on the ply I should pee.

It seemed like a comedy sketch. But it was serious. All went well, and she showed me the read-out on a strip of paper with graduation lines on it. My reading was a trace line down the middle. It didn't mean anything to me, but she was to take it to the next port of call: the urologist.

Dr Shaikh, a really nice chap, told me the result of my PSA test was a reading of 13.7, going on to explain that for someone of my age it should be between 5 and 6, but added that he has patients with numbers in the high hundreds. I had by now convinced myself I had cancer.

The doctor suggested another internal examination. I wasn't prepared for this, and having been walking round town on this hot day before we arrived, I had become a bit sweaty in the trouser department...

Despite this admission, the doctor bravely and selflessly went ahead – only to confirm what the GP had already found. In an involuntary role reversal, I immediately told him that I thought it was cancer. I still remember that moment and his response: 'Whatever it is, it is 100 per cent treatable,' was the reassuring reply, putting my mind completely at ease.

'What do we do next?'

The answer was a bone scan to check that it had not spread;

if it had, it would require a completely different treatment. The bone scan took place exactly two weeks later, in a 'nuclear medicine department'!

A large machine sat in the centre of the scanning room. I was asked to sit in a large swivel chair by the chap in charge, who produced a syringe containing, not the glowing green gloop of my imagination, but about two thimbles' worth of a clear liquid, which he proceeded to inject painlessly, then told me to go away for a couple of hours and drink plenty.

'Will I glow in the dark now?' I asked. He chuckled. 'My daughter wonders whether I'll fart little mushroom clouds.'

This time he laughed out loud. 'That's a new one...'

Hmm. Drink plenty... Down went the bottle of water I'd brought with me. We went into town. Into Greggs for a large coffee. Then Wetherspoons – bowl of chips and a couple of pints of Doom Bar. Time to stagger back up the hill to the hospital.

I kept all my clothes on as I got up on to the machine which, for a change, travelled over me, rather than me travelling through it. This took about 45 minutes, the last ten of which were a bit uncomfortable, as I had to sit on the edge of the bed, dead still in front of a screen scanning my head.

Before leaving I was given a sheet of instructions, including: 'Avoid close contact with pregnant women and small children, drink plenty, pee frequently and flush the toilet twice. Should be back to normal after 24 hours.' I was told to ring the office number on Monday for my results. I phoned the Hemel number: 'Sorry, no one here, they're on holiday.'

I phoned the Watford office: 'Sorry, nobody here to help you. Try St Albans.'

Phoned St Albans: 'Please phone back tomorrow.'

This was the most important result. I needed to know. *Now.* But I had to wait.

Tuesday morning. Phoned St Albans again: 'Sorry, I cannot give information like that over the phone...' I'm afraid I lost it a bit at this point. Explaining my plight, the person at the other end of the line said, 'I'll get back to you.'

Twenty minutes later: 'Mr Arnold? I'm pleased to tell you that the bone scan results are all clear.' Words cannot describe my relief when I heard that.

It was now time to start on hormone treatment. Twenty-eight days of tablets, then three-monthly Decapeptyl injections. So: drugs, blood tests and radiotherapy, the latter starting early in 2019. I was due to continue treatment at Mount Vernon. A 20-mile trip, taking about 40 minutes on average. I began commuting there at the end of January 2019 with a 'programming meeting'.

We arrived, booked in and were seen by a very nice Polish lady and told it would be 45 minutes before I'd be seen and to drink six cups of water. I lost count of the cups, so I had to get rid of as much as possible and start again. The significance of the six cups was to ensure having exactly the same amount of water in your bladder when starting each radiotherapy session.

I was shown into a scanning room with two young women in attendance. Shoes off, jeans off, and I lay on the bed of the machine and kept still. The machine started humming. It wasn't as noisy as the MRI one. I'd only been on it a few minutes when it went quiet. Hmm. That was quick!

Then the two women came in and told me there was a problem. I hadn't emptied my bowel before coming in. To be fair, I hadn't been told to, but apparently the bowel needed to be empty so as not to distort the prostate.

I was given a small plastic tube and sent off to the WC... No, that's not what the tube was for... I was told to break the top off and use the contents as an enema... Nothing more to see here, move on!

It worked... BUT I also allowed some water out... so, back to the drinking before returning for a third attempt to get things right.

I stripped off again. Got back in position, wearing just pants, socks and a T-shirt. Then I heard: 'Ron, could you lower your underwear a bit... NO, NOT THAT FAR!'

I was aware of some giggling going on, but I retrieved my dignity. They placed a square pad, with loads of wires sticking out, over my abdomen and the process began.

'Is that it?'

'No, we now have to tattoo you.'

Radiotherapy started on 5 February at 6.15 pm.

We arrived about two and a half hours early. First thing to do – get car parking sorted, which involved finding the parking office. No mean feat in itself. It was at the end of a long series of corridors. I was given a yellow card to put on the dashboard, entitling me to buy a £1 ticket for each of my 25 visits.

A piece of unexpected advice I was given that day, was to bring a screw-top milk bottle – in case you need it on the way home. This was to do with the effects of drinking water.

We found where we had to go – room LA10 – then had to enter a barcode ticket in a machine to show we had arrived. My turn was not far off.

'Mr Arnold, could you go and drink six cups of water, then come back in.' I managed three cups before my throat went numb. By sipping slowly, I managed the other three. I went back to the waiting room.

'Go and change, please.'

I stripped down to pants, T-shirt and socks. Put on a dressing gown. Stood by the control room door – inside was what resembled the flight deck of the Starship Enterprise. A large room, with a massive machine in the middle, looking like the MRI scanner I'd already used, only somewhat bigger.

Now to climb on to the machine's couch-like table-bed. Two of the staff adjusted a headrest, asked me to raise my knees to put a foam block underneath and then a footrest was placed against my feet.

'Right, Mr Arnold, could you push your pants down a bit, and pull your T-shirt up.' Remembering what happened last time I'd been given similar instructions, I was careful not to overdo the down-ing.

A cloth was placed over my pants and tucked into the waistband. One person either side – they pulled and pushed me into the position they required. A thin, green laser beam shone on to my lower body, with the tattoos used as 'targets'. I had my arms folded across my chest and was told not to move.

They left and the huge door closed. The machine started humming and moving – up, down, around. The whole process lasted about ten minutes, after which there was a click somewhere off to my left and the sound of voices as the girls came back in to lower the bed so that I could disembark – albeit with a paper towel, which they'd left on the bed, becoming entrapped in the back of my pants, and now trailing behind me...

We were now free to go home. I needed a pee before leaving, but five miles from home I was bursting again and had to head for a nearby Shell petrol station – I just about made it, suddenly remembering the advice to carry a screw-top bottle about!

I had 24 appointments remaining. There were none on weekends.

During week two I spotted that the chap ahead of me at the water dispenser pressed a button which read 'room temp' – brilliant, no more struggling with the ice-cold option. On the way home one evening I'd forgotten to empty out before leaving and, down a dark lane, not a moment too soon, I found a use for that screw-top bottle which, it transpired, had an additional use – the car heater was struggling a little, so Jan used the bottle as a hand-warmer.

I took one of the water cups home and worked out that six cups equalled a litre, so I found a litre squash bottle which I filled and brought with me to the waiting room and drank it there.

Having been 'done' we headed off to the canteen – it was in a lovely, high-ceilinged room with large arched windows. The food was brilliant. This pattern also allowed for efficient bladder emptying before departing.

About halfway into the treatment I had a consultation about my waterworks and bowels as radiotherapy can – and often does, apparently – upset both functions. I was asked questions by a charming young lady, including one concerning 'the consistency' of my poo.

I was stumped for an answer before coming up with 'runny with lumps in' which, for some reason, I said in an imitation of the voice of Max Wall. She burst out laughing, which broke the ice, and she then showed me some pictures of poo, so I selected the closest to 'runny with lumps'.

On to the subject of urinary urgency – another common side effect – where she explained pelvic floor exercises and asked me to try for myself, only to start laughing and tell me: 'I don't know what you're doing, Mr Arnold, but raising your shoulders will not help – try moving something a little lower down!'

Around this time, we'd seen a new face in the waiting room, a chap sitting in the corner, wearing a cowboy hat and leather jacket: 'Hello, mate, how're y'doing? Everything going well?'. Told me his name was Graham Sharpe.

It turned out that we had something in common – record collecting! The three of us hit it off and became, and have remained, good friends.

As the treatment came to an end, I noticed that I was getting a little sore 'down there'. I had a chat with one of the technicians about the laser machine – he told me it had cost £1,000,000 from America, and that only the manufacturer could supply spare parts. I was also astonished to discover that a replacement knee support alone cost £2,000 – yet it was effectively just a block covered in plastic.

My final day of radiotherapy felt a bit sad, as we had got to know the team well. The session over, I got dressed and went to say thank you to them. It got a bit emotional. I happened to say to one of the girls, my favourite: 'It must be one of the most rewarding jobs, saving people's lives.' She stunned me by replying that I was one of a very few people who had said that, and she launched herself at me for a really good hug. My eyes were moist, as were hers. Then she reminded me: 'You have got brachytherapy treatment in about a week – these last five weeks have been a walk in the park compared to that.'

I'd had to undertake a check for MRSA [MRSA is a bacteria resistant to some widely-used antibiotics. Also described as a super bug] before undergoing brachytherapy, which involved a short consultation followed by some swabs, one from my nostrils, the other from my groin. I had been advised that, because of the after-effects, I should not drive to the hospital for the brachytherapy, which would begin on 5 March.

Brachytherapy: 'A radiation therapy used as a prostate cancer treatment. Sometimes referred to as interstitial radiation therapy, seed therapy or seed treatment. Prostate brachytherapy is capable of delivering high and concentrated doses of radiation to the prostate gland.'

My neighbour, Wendy, kindly offered to take me. On arrival I trudged off with my overnight bag to ward 10 of Mount Vernon – a ward number which for someone of my age immediately brought to mind the '60s hospital soap opera, *Emergency Ward 10*.

I was booked in, shown my bed and allowed to wander – which I did, to meet the only other occupant, although another soon arrived. This was Murray, a London fireman of similar age and sense of humour to me, here for the same reason. I then delivered some chocolates and biscuits to the radiography team in LA10 where they were, as usual, in full swing.

Back at ward 10 there was a blood test, a blood pressure check, a kind of ECG and a request for a urine sample to be supplied in a grey bottle. I provided the sample, put the grey bottle on the table tray and told the nurse, repeating the message an hour later.

I'd requested a sandwich and some juice for tea time, which were put on my tray next to the grey bottle. I didn't fancy having it there while I was eating, so I moved it to the floor. Once I'd finished I moved the tray, and inevitably knocked over the grey bottle in the process, spilling its contents over the floor. I then had to provide a second sample, taken away much more quickly.

At around 10 pm two nurses arrived: 'Time for your enema, Mr Arnold.'

I was ready for this and asked where the funnel, rubber tube and bucket of soapy water were... The nurses laughed. 'This is the twenty-first century, Mr Arnold!' One of the nurses then produced what looked like a small tube of toothpaste, telling me to lay on my right side, first pulling down my pyjama trousers, then pulling my knees up to my chest. She snapped the top off the tube, which had a longish nozzle, shoved it in my anus and squeezed out the contents.

Twenty-five minutes later: 'Gotta go!'

It was intense, and as it was so warm in there I nearly passed out. Back in bed I was given some tablets to stop any further bowel movements. I had a last drink and a couple of biscuits, as I was to be nil by mouth from midnight, and tried to sleep. Sleep? Murray was snoring as though he'd taken a chainsaw to bed, and on the other side the chap had some sort of machine running all night. Not a wink of sleep did I get, so 7.30 am came as a relief when I was told to take a shower.

Back at base camp I was presented with a fashionable hospital gown, from which it was impossible to prevent one's rear end from protruding, and a strange little packet, which turned out to contain socks – but not as we know them – which had a hole at the end so that your toes poked through and were so tight as to be almost impossible to tug on. Pressure socks, apparently.

Two porters arrived... but went straight past me, up to the far end of the ward where, unbeknown to us, another patient had arrived, residing behind a partition wall. He appeared in a wheelchair and was taken away by the porters, who brought him back nearly an hour later, with tubes coming out of him and up into two containers which were full of clear liquid, and suspended above the trolley bed he was lying on. Then the porters came for Murray. 'Good luck, mate,' I called. 'See you soon.'

Fifty minutes later he was back, now in a similar condition to the newcomer, and was slid on to the bed. He didn't seem to be moving but was soon chatting.

I remembered we'd been told we would have to lay still on our backs for some seven hours because of the implants – if we moved, we ran the risk of displacing them. I asked Murray: 'What was it like?'

He laughed. 'Different.'

It was soon my turn. Dentures went into a pot on the bedside cupboard, along with my glasses and watch; I went into the wheelchair, blankets wrapped around me, and off I went with a 'Good luck!' from Murray ringing in my ears.

I was soon appreciating the blankets as we reached the main entrance and went outside – it was bloody freezing and blowing a gale. Into the back of an ambulance I went, and although I'm still not sure where it travelled, we couldn't have been that far away as we were soon going through the doors of another building, into a lift and up to a room where I was transferred on to a trolley.

Two nurses appeared. One proceeded to insert a canular into the back of my right hand, fitted a syringe and pushed the plunger. A male voice began talking from behind my bed, asking me about my favourite holiday resort... I got as far as saying, 'Sennen Cove, near L... a... n... d... s... E... n...', before I was gone.

Next thing – although it wasn't, really – I felt a mask on my face, then heard a nurse asking how I was. 'Light-headed' was the truth... and I was realising that something was a bit weird down in the trouser department. Not to mention the strange tubes and liquid containers looming over me... The following hours remain a bit of a blur. I was on my back for six or seven of them and saw an awful lot of ceiling.

The next port of call was for a CT scan. Then back to the ward to compare notes with Murray. Later, another CT scan to make sure my 'applicators' had not budged. Applicators were, I was told, needles, and in my case I had 21 applicators inserted through my perineum and into the prostate. I was told that I had to have an extra one to cap a lymph node which was also infected.

All of this equipment was inserted under general anaesthetic, as was the catheter, of which, more later...

I also had an MRI scan which was where I got some earplugs from, because the scanner was noisy. I kept these and scrounged another pair – which I later gave to the staff of ward 10, who told me they had a job getting a supply for their own patients.

The porters were back a couple of hours later. I was transferred from bed to trolley. Tricky, given that I was still not allowed to move myself. Hands across my chest, wrapped in a blanket, rolled on one side. A fabric sheet with handles on either side had been laid on the bed. I was rolled back onto this sheet and, via the handles, slid on to the trolley.

Into the treatment room. Squeamish readers should look away now. Legs bent, knees as far apart as possible. A strange movement felt as the doctor adjusted the needles. No pain, but a weird sensation as he moved the prostate by 'tweaking' the needles.

Once he was satisfied, I was off to a different area of the room for treatment apparently involving connecting a coded wire to the exposed end of each needle – the pointy ends of which contained tiny 'seeds' of radioactive material.

Once this was done, the doctor and a nurse went to the control panel behind a glass screen and began to 'switch me on'. This took about 20 minutes. I lost track of time. There was no sensation whatsoever. Now, for the next bit of action!

I'm lying there, legs bent, knees apart, hospital gown serving no useful purpose. I hear female voices and raise my head – three ladies were staring intently at my exposed undercarriage.

'Right, Mr Arnold, we are going to remove the needles.' One at a time. No pain, just a slight pulling sensation.

After a couple of minutes, they told me that about a third around the outside of the area had been removed, and that I now had a choice... 'We can remove the remainder individually, or... pull them out in one go...'

'Er... ok... go for it!'

'Take a deep breath...'

I was halfway through the inhale, then... 'BLOODY HELL!'

But that was it, about a second and they were out. A hand

immediately shoved a large wad of tissue over the area, there was a bit of a clean-up and I was soon safely back in bed in ward 10.

I was allowed to sit up and move – bliss. Glasses on, teeth in, watch on. I was able to eat and drink which I hadn't done for some 18 hours. The cup of tea was like nectar, and I finished all the biscuits I'd brought with me.

Our 'Trolley Dolly' gave me the menu for the evening meal. I've kept it. Whatever you have heard about hospital food – forget it. The food was excellent. White roll and butter. Cream of chicken soup. Lamb and mint pie. Mashed spuds, mixed veg. All washed down with orange juice. Ice cream and mixed fruit to follow.

The evening staff arrived, amongst them Julia, a tall, 40-something Irish lady with, it turned out, a wicked sense of humour. It was a really funny evening – non-stop laughter for three hours – my mate and I agreed that it was the tonic we needed after the day we'd had. At one stage, there were some six members of staff round our beds – a young, black, male nurse was laughing so much that he only just stopped himself from falling over. Then there came the time for sleep; I had earplugs ready.

We were plugged into two-litre containers of clear liquid, which was saline solution for irrigation – gravity forced the liquid to flow into the catheter, then it went into the bladder and out and down a second tube into a clear plastic bag hanging by the side of the bed. This procedure – which continued all night, featuring fresh bottles of saline and changed bags – was to help heal and flush out any blood, etc, which might be in the waterworks. The bag changing produced some amusing comments: 'That's a cherryade', 'Yes, a nice rosé'. In the early hours when I was half awake, I heard: 'A half-decent chardonnay, nearly there.' When I later heard 'gin' and 'vodka', I knew I must be there!

I was awakened by someone tapping on my shoulder at about 7.30 am. What was she saying to me? Had I gone deaf? No, you dopey old sod, I chastised myself, you've got earplugs in! Once removed, I heard: 'Morning, Ron – time to take the catheter out. Swing your legs over the edge of the bed.'

Legs pressed slightly apart, tubes removed from bottles and bag. Only a tube protruding from inside me was left. The nurse grabbed hold of the end of it and slowly began to pull... Erm, how much more is there? I thought. It was well over a foot long, with a flattened end. Probably best not to know how it was originally inserted...

Now I was told that I could go home... once I had shown that I could poo and pee normally.

Grey-bottle time produced a small amount of liquid, and I was told to drink plenty of water – so that next time there was a better flow. That'll do it, I told myself.

Except that when I double checked there was only a damp patch and a large puddle on the floor – there was a hole in my bottle!

Annoyed, I had to start again – once I'd got the sock-things off – which was at least as difficult as putting the blooming things on. Drink water, pee, drink more water, pee – I had a big incentive to do this, having been warned that if I didn't produce enough, I'd have to wear a catheter for a further fortnight.

Murray came up with an idea – take the bottle to the washroom, run a tap, and hope the sound helped prompt a healthy flow. It worked for him. But not for me. However, having checked that there was no one around, I just topped the bottle up from the tap, whilst admittedly still worrying whether, if they analysed it, they would wonder why there was chlorine in my sample...

Anyway, I was given the okay to go home. A quick call sorted a lift. Before that I discovered why my bed was a little uncomfortable. When the porters had brought me back the previous day, they'd left that thing with the handles in it... Time to tidy up and have a final chat with Murray. We said our farewells, wished each other well, and he was gone.

I had written a card and brought in some chocs and biscuits to say thanks to the team – I gave the bag to one of the staff, Cassie, who jokingly pretended to run off with it, but then came over for a big hug.

That was about that. No serious after-effects, other than being a little sore for a couple of days. I had a salt bath at home and found that I was as black as the ace of spades where the needles had been.

I was put on three-monthly hormone treatment – injections of Decapeptyl into the buttocks, alternate buttocks at each visit. These jabs have done certain things to my body – for starters, my nuts have nearly disappeared. I think they have migrated up my chest and tried to turn into boobs. Then there's the hot flushes – okay during the winter, not so much fun during summer – but don't expect any sympathy from ladies of a certain age when you tell them.

I've also experienced some weight gain in my lower stomach area, but all in all a small price to pay.

***

Ron and I have stayed in touch on a regular basis during the pandemic. I believe we both feel we can be more honest and open with each other because of what we went, and came, through together.

A month or so after both of our treatments had finished, I read this in the *Daily Mail* on 29 April 2019 (Sheila's birthday):

The findings, presented at the European Society for Radiotherapy and Oncology conference in Milan, suggest that... a single blast of radiotherapy could save prostate cancer patients weeks of gruelling treatment... ...researchers, from the Christie hospital in Manchester and Mount Vernon in London, found all men with low-risk cancer were clear of the disease three years after receiving the treatment, which usually takes just ten to 20 minutes... High dose-rate brachytherapy – which delivers a powerful surge of radiotherapy direct to the prostate in one single session – is safe and effective for men with low-risk cancer, researchers found.

Such treatment would also lessen the risk of side effects and reduce the toxic impact to surrounding healthy tissue. Some patients with medium and high-risk PC were also successfully treated.

16

IN WHICH I TALK TO A STILL GRIEVING PROSTATE WIDOW

WRITING ABOUT PC has forced me to confront the brutal truth – that although many appear to have come through their treatment successfully and have been handed an enhanced future... the risk of a relapse, or the hammer blow of discovering that the old symptoms remain – or that new, but equally, if not more, dangerous ones emerge – is always hovering above and around PC patients. The disease is equally threatening to 'normal' blokes as it is to world-famous sporting superstars. As Lauren, the wife of England cricketer Bob Willis, discovered.

Bob Willis, one of the greatest fast bowlers and biggest characters ever to grace the sport of cricket, died of PC on 4 December 2019. He was a little over halfway through his 71st year. Bob's sporting immortality was ensured by his and Ian Botham's heroics in an amazing turn-round victory over deadly enemies, the Aussies, in the 1981 Headingley Test Match, in which they were quoted during the match at 500/1 to win, only for Bob's legendary 8-43 bowling and Ian Botham's innings of 149 to swing the game.

There was shock and an outpouring of emotional tributes for the player, who had not wanted to publicise his situation, when news of Bob's death broke. Lauren, who met him initially through her career in sports publishing and TV before they became a couple in 2005, told me how Bob's illness had affected her: 'Bob was just stoic and accepting of it. He never complained once during the whole time, he was very brave, took everything onboard. We just carried on having fun. For nearly three and a half years, he wasn't too bad really and then it was a very, very sudden demise at the end.

Bob had had a few urinary tract infections over the past few years, but had first gone to the doctor with a UTI in early January. Were they suggesting there was something else going on? He took a PSA test – they can be unreliable and a low PSA count does not guarantee that there is no cancer – which produced a reading of 7. He went to see an NHS urologist who told him in so many words that he could assure him he had nothing to worry about but told him to come back in six weeks.'

Lauren and Bob decided to take a pre-booked holiday to California's Napa Valley, where Bob was keen to learn more about, and indulge in one of his major interests – wine. 'Bob's PSA was 6.2, and he had already had the biopsy by the time we went to America in April 2016. We got the results when we came back on April 20.'

Bob was told his 'Gleason score', which indicated the seriousness of the condition was very high. Nine out of ten. 'It was appalling,' Lauren said in an interview with the *Mail on Sunday*'s medical editor, Stephen Adams: 'Appalling that there had obviously been signs that he might have cancer, and appalling that it took three months from the PSA test to knowing he had it.'

**The Gleason score and Grade Groups

The Gleason score is the most common system doctors use to grade prostate cancer. The grade of a cancer tells you how much the cancer cells look like normal cells. This gives your doctor an idea of how the cancer might behave and what treatment you need.

To find out the Gleason score or Grade Group, a pathologist looks at several samples of cells (biopsies) from your prostate.

The pathologist grades each sample of prostate cancer cells from 3 to 5 based on how quickly they are likely to grow or how aggressive the cells look. You may hear this score being called the Gleason Grade.

Doctors then work out an overall Gleason score by adding together the 2 most common Gleason grades. So for example, if the most common Gleason grade is 3, and the second most common is 4, then the overall Gleason score is 7. Or they might write the scores separately as 3 + 4 = 7. This combined score is also now called the Grade Group.

There are 5 Grade Groups. Grade Group 1 is the least aggressive and Grade Group 5 is the most aggressive.

This is how the Gleason score and Grade Groups match up and what it means:

Gleason score	Grade Group	What it means
Gleason score 6 (or 3 + 3 = 6)	Grade Group 1	The cells look similar to normal prostate cells. The cancer is likely to grow very slowly, if at all
Gleason score 7 (or 3 + 4 = 7)	Grade Group 2	Most cells still look similar to normal prostate cells. The cancer is likely to grow slowly
Gleason score 7 (or 4 + 3 = 7)	Grade Group 3	The cells look less like normal prostate cells. The cancer is likely to grow at a moderate rate

Gleason score	Grade Group	What it means
Gleason score 8 (or 4 + 4 = 8)	Grade Group 4	Some cells look abnormal. The cancer might grow quickly or at a moderate rate
Gleason score 9 or 10 (or 4 + 5 = 9, 5 + 4 = 9 or 5 + 5 = 10)	Grade Group 5	The cells look very abnormal. The cancer is likely to grow quickly

**Information from the Cancer Research UK website.

'Bob hadn't had any idea the outcome may be that high,' Lauren wrote to me. 'I didn't go to any of his earliest appointments. I had had a friend who died from prostate cancer. I was hoping it could be something not so serious. This was the worst possible scenario which could indicate a remaining lifespan of six months. But Bob would live for another three years and eight months.'

Bob himself explained how the news of his cancer diagnosis, in April 2016, affected him. He liaised with *Daily Mail* journalist and close friend, Mike Dickson, in May 2019, when they were planning a new autobiography.

Bob wrote: 'I recall being reasonably stoic upon hearing the news, although it did feel something akin to sustaining a huge blow to the solar plexus. I was stunned for the next two or three hours, until I started to come to terms with what I had been told. Nor did I feel much in the way of self-pity, although you inevitably ask yourself why it is you whose number has come up.'

'We were worried. [We] felt sick,' recalled Lauren in her email. 'On the day Bob was diagnosed we read a piece in the paper about prostate cancer and chicken, which was, according to this piece, really bad for prostate cancer. We'd eaten a lot of chicken but immediately gave it up. I still don't eat meat now. We bought a book called *How Not to Die*.' Lauren continued: 'He didn't moan, he never felt sorry for himself, he never cried. And, unfortunately, we didn't really talk about him dying, because I think when you're so close to it all, you don't realise what's happening and no one was actually saying he's dying.'

Until just three months before he died, Bob was still appearing on Sky TV giving his cricketing opinions, was still socialising with friends and playing the occasional round of golf. Because of his television commitments, Lauren had been insistent that Bob should wear a 'cold cap' while he was undergoing treatments including chemotherapy injections, to stop his hair falling out: 'I didn't want him looking like a cancer victim.'

She was successful in this aim and even Bob's consultant oncologist Dr Lisa Pickering said, 'I saw him on television knowing he was on chemo. He definitely lived longer because of it, and it enabled him to keep working.' But when the end came it was brutally sudden. This from the *Daily Mail*: '"I wasn't expecting it at all... Two days before he died, he wanted to go to work," says Lauren.'

'So, it was a major shock really, and by the time I really knew he was dying, he was asleep. That's a bit sad that we didn't... there was a moment where I said to him when he was still at home, "It's not much fun this, is it?"

He looked at me really seriously and said, "No." So, that was about the only sort of moment we actually thought about what was happening. I don't want to have any regrets, I don't think that I could have done anything else – having a horrible conversation about dying – I don't know how useful that would have been anyway.'

He died at a private hospital in Wimbledon as 'Positively Fourth Street', his favourite track by his idol Bob Dylan – he'd even added Dylan to his own name by deed poll – was playing.

'People seem to really miss Bob,' Lauren reflected, 'I mean, every day on social media, there's stuff about him. After he died, it was a bit of the "David Bowie of the cricketing world" type "wow" moment, because viewers had only recently seen him on telly. He would not have believed the outpouring of grief. To me he seems more famous now than when he was alive.'

Of course, it is the person left behind who then has to come to terms with an entirely new approach to their life, and that is even more difficult when there is also a pandemic to cope with as well, and you are living on your own:

'We did everything together all the time, we were a team. Bob was my best friend, all those usual clichés. And now, suddenly, I'm living on my own for the first time in my whole life and it isn't very helpful that the Covid-19 lockdown has been going on and really isolating me. I'm handling it most days okay, I've been painting pictures of Bob's bowling action, but I feel like I'm nobody's priority anymore. Post Covid, I don't really know what my life consists of when I get through it. All I really want at the moment is to be able to socialise and hug people, because you miss all that. You just suddenly maybe can never, ever even have a hug again, I mean, it's hideous because of the Covid side – really, really tough.'

Lauren wanted a call to action, to encourage others to support Prostate Cancer UK. She and Bob's brother, David, remain supportive, whilst launching, and now working for, their own Bob Willis Fund.

'I want to help people with it. I want Bob to have a legacy, you know, I want to think about him all the time, so that's really why Bob's brother, David, and I are both so keen to support Prostate Cancer UK. There are a lot of things to be done about it, and no time to waste.

I would love to see an improved blood test, more accurate than the PSA test, that determines the severity of prostate cancer much quicker, so that men and [their] families can understand sooner how aggressive or otherwise their disease is.

I think the PSA probably is accurate for a lot of men, but it wasn't accurate for Bob. You can have a high PSA reading that suggests there's something going on, and you can have a PSA that's low and yet it's really advanced aggressive prostate cancer. We clearly need a better test than that.'

I first spoke to Lauren in mid-October 2020 during the pandemic, when London was in the middle tier of a three-tier 'lockdown' system. Lauren was living on her own:

'It isn't easy. I've never lived on my own before. It is hard to take on board. Everything which might help me recover following Bob's death it seems I can't do.'

She told me about Bob's treatment experiences: 'I went with him to an appointment at St George's, Tooting, where the oncologist suggested three-monthly injections, together with PSA tests. A nurse said to Bob: "You're having chemo." His experiences here were a total shambles thanks to the attitude of the male consultant he was seeing.

We were told about a consultant named Dr Lisa Pickering, who did private work, and was then based at the Cancer Centre in Wimbledon. I loved her. She was the only good thing to come out of this whole situation.

I got on really well with her and she insisted we needed to do everything through her. July 11, 2016 was when she first began treating Bob, with his first round of DTX (Docetaxel). He had six rounds of treatment with three monthly injections.

Every single treatment seemed to help, but didn't seem to last long-term. Bob was very upfront about having the chemotherapy, and we never discussed how long it would go on for. Bob probably didn't want to know. However, he went along with everything I wanted him to do. I was so reassuringly vital to him towards the end. He wanted me to be there all the time.

To think that now, during the pandemic, maybe I now wouldn't have been allowed to go to hospital with him. I wanted to keep his situation private. His main nurse during treatment was hilarious. She'd say, "Come on, let's get this done so we can have Cheltenham on the TV and put some bets on." As soon as the session was finished, Bob wanted to get to a pub to have a beer, to make it all a more acceptable part of everyday life.

I felt this should all remain private. I didn't want to see a headline scrolling across Sky News screens that "Bob Willis has Prostate Cancer".

When it became evident the chemo wasn't working he had some strong radiotherapy. We couldn't sleep in the same bed for a week during this, and it buggered up his blood. Ultimately his white blood cell count went so low that I think we accepted he was going to die.

He had a very horrible time at the end. Peeing eight times a night, which resulted in having to have a catheter.

Bob was in hospital for thirty days of the final ten weeks of his life. They tried a final chemo session. Eventually we'd begun to tell people – initially his daughter, friends and bosses at Sky. They all kept it as private as possible.

Since Bob died I've been doing a lot of publicity for PC UK. On the Adrian Chiles show I was able to mention some of his side effects. I think it should be more widely understood. I understand that a lot of men are reluctant to tell their mates – particularly if they're Aussies like many of Bob's – that they can no longer "have a shag". It can be awful for the person to suffer shrunken testicles and penis, and loss of sexual appetite.

But it is now the number one cancer from which men suffer. There are, of course, other symptoms I was upset with myself for not mentioning, such as the difficulties with peeing, the ordeal of a biopsy, which are not very nice.'

By the time I spoke to Lauren, she had ramped up her thoughts and was considering launching the Bob Willis Foundation: 'I want the Bob Willis Foundation to raise money for prostate cancer and nothing else (at this point). I want people to know when you say Bob Willis Foundation it means for prostate cancer research.' She already knew what she wanted it to stand for.

'This is the message I want to get across:

"The Bob Willis Foundation was formed in memory of the legendary former England Cricket Captain who died of Prostate Cancer in 2019 aged just 70.

Prostate Cancer is now the most commonly diagnosed of all cancers in the UK and improvements need to be made in the testing and diagnosis process. The PSA blood test can be a useful indicator in a lot of men, but it wasn't accurate enough for Bob.

The Bob Willis Foundation aims to raise awareness and money to help develop a better test to determine the severity of the disease much quicker. It's a very serious disease that can be deadly. We need to find treatments and tests that will help men like Bob in the future."'

Launching the Foundation (later to become the Bob Willis Fund) struck me as an excellent idea, and also chimed with thoughts I'd been having about the difficulty for a PC patient in knowing where to look for up-to-date information about the latest treatments and research concerning PC.

Of course, newspapers will often write pieces about such developments, but unless you read every paper and website every day you won't be able to keep abreast of everything. Googling 'prostate cancer' can take you off into all sorts of highways and byways of information – genuine, iffy, unreliable, baffling, authoritative – with no real quality control around to advise you whether what you're reading is credible or crazy, or whether it is designed to enlighten you or to lighten your pocket by taking advantage of your vulnerability when you are suffering from a disease.

I contacted Prostate Cancer UK's head of brand and media, Phil Wye, to discover his organisation's thoughts and he responded in depth:

Thanks for dropping us a line at Prostate Cancer UK, and as you're a man who's been affected by the disease I hope you're doing well at this time.

You're right to point out that via our website we demonstrate the work we're funding and the impact we've made, rather than catalogue all ongoing research.

To your enquiry – is there, or might there be, a one-stop shop with regards to prostate cancer research? In truth there's a vast range of global sources, stretching far beyond what would be feasible for us as a UK charity to invest resources in collating and storing. Across the globe, some research varies widely from others.

For clinical trials there's **clinicaltrials.gov** which is comprehensive (it's driven by the fact that all trials need to have a registration number).

Part of the value of our team of research staff is that by attending conferences that gives them the best way to get sight of loads of ongoing research which they report back on.

In terms of results – https://pubmed.ncbi.nlm.nih.gov/ is the go-to for pretty much all papers published. But it's not tailored for a public audience so much.

So that's essentially an answer for you, and I hope it's helpful.

A bit more on our work:

Our strategic approach is to support the research that our experts believe has the greatest potential for change, conducted by the best researchers, and guided by a rigorous funding policy.

We fund leading research by using innovative approaches and continuing to meet the Association of Medical Research Charities' guidance on best practice in research funding.

By monitoring and evaluating the outcomes of our research, we use the knowledge we gain to best effect, either by funding further research or by supporting translation into clinical practice.

We foster a flourishing prostate cancer research environment in the UK and supporting the next generation of leading prostate cancer researchers.

Please know that we are evidence-led:

By learning from, and acting on, research in other diseases, countries and funders.

By actively contributing to the acquisition of new knowledge about prostate cancer, and using this to constantly evolve our approach to research.

By using what we learn from new, big data approaches to guide and inform our future research priorities.

We partner for the most impact:

With men affected by prostate cancer, their families, partners and carers to ensure they stay at the heart of our work.

With international experts in research, data collection and analysis, and the delivery of prostate cancer treatment and care.

With other research funders across the world and other interested stakeholders who can help to ensure that research results are put into practice.

Stay safe, very best regards,

Phil...

Head of Brand & Media
Prostate Cancer UK

When I shared Phil's response with Lauren, she declared:

That's a pretty detailed response from Phil. He's my favourite guy to deal with there. I suppose, in reality, nobody is really interested in knowing about detailed research until you are diagnosed and then you become very interested.

Then you hope your doctor knows all about it. During Bob's treatment there were lots of positive messages coming from conferences in Chicago. And as you say there are often pieces in papers about brilliant new treatments that they say can extend your life by about two months!

Because Bob was "private" he'd usually already tried these treatments before they hit the papers.

I have known Bob's brother, David, for a good number of years, initially as a result of both of us being involved with major annual prizes for the best sports books published in the UK.

Of course, David was devastated by his brother's passing, and when we spoke, he told me that he and a couple of close cricketing friends of Bob's – international players – had recently gathered together to mark the first anniversary of his death, and to raise a glass to him. They, and others he had consulted, had all agreed they would like to support David's efforts to create a fundraising 'Blue for Bob' day in the cricket calendar, which was already resulting in big names of the sport pledging their support.

As a result of Bob's situation, David had made sure to get himself checked out regularly, and agrees with his sister-in-law, Lauren, that one of the most important directions for funding to go towards is improving early diagnosis for those potentially at risk – something which is still somewhat hit and miss at the moment.

'I understand that the prostate gland can be a magnet for cancer cells,' David noted. He continued:

In Bob's case he had them in a hip and a rib, and they can spread into the major organs, leading to fatal results. So, anything we can do to improve early diagnosis and treatment will be invaluable.

We don't want to raise money only for it to disappear into a general sinkhole and believe that whatever we can raise should be directed towards early diagnosis, particularly after discovering some sobering statistics, such as that one man dies on average every 45 minutes of prostate cancer, and that in every cricket match taking place it is likely that two or three of those taking part could end up getting prostate cancer.

And of course, this alarming statistic can also be applied to other sports such as football and rugby.

17

IN WHICH MY BEST MATE SHOWS HIS CLASS

NOW, LET me introduce you to the false sense of euphoria that I - and, I guess, many others - experienced when the radiotherapy sessions ended... only to remember all too vividly that I'd been warned that the treatment is accumulative, and that its effects can linger for weeks more.

I'd known that the urination and diarrhoea could remain with me, but I felt that returning to ordinary life might reveal whether or not some of these were psychological rather than physical effects. So I took myself off for a haircut, my first since beginning treatment.

Karl, my barber, initially pretended he didn't recognise me, then took a closer look and said, 'You've lost weight.' During the natural course of our conversation, he told me that his daughter was working in the radiotherapy department at Mount V.

Should I tell him? I thought to myself. But by now he was well into some of his favourite angling tales and had stopped fishing for info about my absence, so I was off the hook. I came out less hairy and relieved that I hadn't had to relieve myself.

But the situation deteriorated and within a few days I felt I had to ring the Mount V radiography department for reassurance. I was reassured - if reassurance was to be told that this sounded par for the course, and that I might wish to invest in some underwear pads to avoid embarrassment... I was also told to keep drinking a couple of litres of water a day, but to ring back if the symptoms 'persisted'. They did. And I still had diarrhoea as well.

My treatment had definitely brought Sheila and I closer together - I mean, after 45 years of marriage we were pretty close already, but she was the only one I felt comfortable confiding in about all of the symptoms. She's far too good-hearted for me and I know I have always been happier keeping my true feelings to myself, which can't be a healthy situation – although I do blame my equally buttoned-up mum for imbuing that attitude in me. No reason I couldn't have chosen to ignore it, mind you.

I was still having to get up several times a night and now had a receptacle by my bed to urinate into, awaking one morning to notice that I'd let the arm of a jumper I'd been wearing dangle into the bucket... I had to surreptitiously wash and tumble dry it without Sheila suspecting anything.

I was by now convinced I had some form of radiotherapy-induced cystitis. I called Mount V and was told to bring in a sample. However, I had also lost confidence in going out at all for fear of being caught short. How was I going to make it to Mount V with a sample bottle without ending up damp?

I decided I had to ask my best mate if he'd give me a lift and to confess the reason to him once we were en route. Like the reliable friend he's always been, Graham Brown agreed immediately – before I'd told him any reason – and said he'd be round at 9 am the next morning, 4 April, to pick me up.

When I told him, he batted not an eyelid, insisted on paying the car-parking fee and waiting with me while I was seen – thus becoming, albeit temporarily, an honorary LA10-er. I saw a radiographer guy called Guy who reassured me that my symptoms were commonplace – no one had really warned me of this, I reflected – and only to be expected. As I was explaining this to Graham, a charming young lady entered the waiting room and began chatting to us. She remains the only person I've ever seen wearing those trainers which have individual toe-shaped apertures at the front in which one inserts one's toes. She assured us these were 'the most comfy' trainers she'd ever owned before revealing a rather more serious secret – she'd been out with her husband when he touched a tiny lump in her neck, which turned out to be escalating into cancer. She'd been off work for a year, but was now able to return to some of her duties, although she was here for a 20-session radiotherapy treatment. Her hair was thin, but, if you'd met her away from the hospital you'd have had no reason to think she looked unwell.

The radiographer guy, Guy, arrived to collect a sample from me – although it took him longer to find a container than it did for me to fill it to overflowing (once you start when you're in this condition it is very difficult to halt the flow) with unpleasantly thick, very yellow, urine. Guy took it off to examine, returning to say he'd found some blood in it and wanted to send it off for further investigation. He'd have to notify me of the results in a couple of days.

Oddly, my euphoria at having completed my radiotherapy seemed to be wearing off... rapidly. Maybe a new pair of toed trainers would help.

Graham returned me home. We shook hands (yes, that's how long ago this happened) and I told him I had no problem with him telling his wife, Anita. I then learnt that Anita had apparently, very recently on a day trip to Brighton, rescued the landlord of the pub where they'd gone for lunch – who had somehow got superglue on himself and begun to panic – by showing him how to sort it with salt and water. 'He was so excited he forgot to buy her a thank you drink,' remembered Graham.

Now I had to deal with the absolute, wretched despair of suffering a UTI, when I'd instinctively built up my hopes that I was on the way back to full health, only to find myself confined to home, becoming over familiar with the bathroom and its toilet... For that same reason I would later have to stay at home in early April, when Sheila and friends went off to a gig.

The next day I was at the dental surgery to have a crown replaced – six hundred and fifty quid, if you please! When I arrived home, I had a call from Mount V, telling me that my urine test showed I had cystitis-like symptoms and that this was something only to be expected after radiotherapy.

I found myself wrestling with the difficulties of avoiding going to the toilet every couple of hours, whilst still keeping myself hydrated and practising my pelvic floor exercises... and wondering how likely this situation was to persist permanently... I took a chance by attending the monthly quiz night for which we had formed a team, and only had to go once during the evening, although ended up scampering home to safety at the end. Graham and I had bumped into each other in a corridor during the quiz and he said quietly to me: 'Thanks for telling me all that.' We shook hands again.

The next day I really wasn't up to going to a concert I had booked tickets for, so I had to let Sheila go with the friends who were coming with us.

With our trip to San Francisco still in doubt, I decided I'd better get used to submitting myself to yet another indignity, and actually put on a pair of absorbent pants. Despite this I didn't feel confident enough to go and watch a Luton home game, and instead stayed indoors on what was Grand National day. No, I didn't back the winner, mine unseated its rider as Tiger Roll won for the second straight year.

Despite now being ten days out from having finished radiotherapy, I was still having to dash to the bathroom on numerous occasions per day, sometimes for diarrhoea-relieving reasons. To make matters worse, my imminent crown space's temporary filling lived up to its billing and fell out. I wasn't due back there for a fortnight. That's if I survived that long.

I tried another tactic designed to keep my mind occupied, hoping that might permit me some increased time between bathroom visits – I went out to pick up litter around the green in our road, attempting to do three circuits before returning.

I completed the three, coming back with crushed cans, discarded paper bags, cardboard, sweet wrappers etc, to be dropped in the bin, only to find myself rushing to the bathroom and wetting myself in the process...

Two weeks on from the end of radiotherapy, I was in my doc's surgery, fortunately seen promptly to hand over a urine sample, as he prescribed some antibiotic tablets to be collected later. He'd had no update from Mount V, so he wasn't even aware I'd finished the radiotherapy course. He didn't warn me to cancel the US trip but did offer to provide an explanatory note if we decided to abandon it, to help with a refund via insurance.

Back indoors I had to go again – this time seeing more blood appearing. Dr K had told me to stay hydrated as much as possible. He advised me to stick to drinking de-caff tea, but also to contact a Macmillan urological nurse, which I did, and her advice was certainly reassuring that this wouldn't remain a permanent state of affairs.

I began taking the pills with my gourmet lunch of baked beans on toast... the next day I attended lunch at quite a posh restaurant, along with my wife, my younger brother and his wife, and my slightly younger sister. I was going to have to tell them about my situation.

The restaurant, I was quick to discover, boasted a fine gents' facility. I was now into my second day of antibiotics and I was hoping their effect would be starting to show.

I broke the news to my fellow family members and, as I suspected would be the case, they were all appropriately sympathetic, but the revelation elicited a suggestion from my brother that our dad may have had some form of cancer treatment. I didn't remember hearing about anything of that nature, though that certainly would not preclude the possibility. Ours was a family in which medical matters were barely referred to in general conversation, although at family parties involving uncles, aunts and cousins one would regularly hear all kinds of unsubstantiated rumours which might or might not contain a kernel of truth.

Returning home, I continued my experiment of seeing how many times I could walk round the green without having to sprint back indoors to relieve myself. This made the book I was reading by Phil Hewitt – *Outrunning the Demons*, about individuals facing various life crises by running sometimes extraordinary distances to help deal with their situations – seem like a panacea I could not currently even contemplate.

The next morning, Saturday, 13 April, I received a text from my

GP informing me that I'd been prescribed the wrong antibiotic and telling me that the correct prescription could be collected from the surgery on Monday.

Oh, so THAT'S why I'd seen virtually no improvement! There was no indication, though, of whether I should continue with the pills I had left or chuck them away. He hadn't said to do the latter, so I continued taking them. I know, I know...

There was no overnight improvement, and I noticed Sheila was looking tired and drained. She had been doing a lot of worrying on my behalf, I was pretty sure. We could both really do with this San Francisco sojourn, but would I be in any position to take it?

I was pinning all my hopes on the Monday medication and rushed down to the doc's to claim my new prescription, but the receptionist could find no trace of it, despite a double check. I explained what had happened and showed her the text. She was also dealing with an 85-year-old begging for Co-codamol tablets, but I pulled rank and demanded my prescription, which then had to be signed by another doctor.

Whilst waiting for this saga to play out, a local friend walked into the surgery. 'Oh,' he said, 'How are you?'

'Stephen, we're both in a doctor's surgery, how do you THINK I am!?'

He replied: 'I'm here for a prescription for my wife.'

'You need a prescription to get a wife?'

I was finally handed my scrip and dashed back to the pharmacy. 'Take three a day with water – throw the others away,' I was told. After a quick trip into Morrisons to grab some shopping, I took the first tablet, accompanied by a hot cross bun, because I'd noticed in the small print on the pill container that to avoid a sickness side effect the pill should be accompanied by food. That afternoon I rang Ashleigh at the travel agency to tell her that we may have to postpone the holiday.

On Tuesday, 16 April I became a great uncle, as my niece Cassie produced a 7lb 6oz boy, Harvey. I also had to calm down my stressed wife as our brand-new washing machine went rogue.

A confirmatory call from the travel agent stating that, yes, we could delay our holiday, included a mumbled subclause which I had to ask her to repeat. Yes, I had heard correctly. It would cost £687 to make the change. About the cost of a new-new washing machine! We would now depart in late May.

With close family and best mate informed of my condition, I knew others should eventually, albeit probably sooner rather than later, be told. I thought I'd wait until antibiotic rescue – I hoped – came galloping over the hill.

The travel agent told me she'd softened the cancellation cost blow, by getting us complimentary tickets to see Alcatraz. 'Does it still have working toilets?' I asked. I'd now taken a third of the tablets.

On Good Friday, I spotted clots in my urine, and desperately hoped they might be evidence of my infection being purged out of me.

On Easter Saturday I was able to survive a three-hour stint without rushing to the bathroom in the morning, then I went to a football match in the afternoon – again managing a three-hour gap, and repeated the feat in the evening. At last, a positive day. Sheila's ongoing support enhanced my feeling that just maybe this was at least the beginning of the end...

The next day I dared to visit a record fair, my first for many months. I held out without going until returning home, where I unleashed a bloody mixture of discoloured fluids and gunge which I hoped was the detritus from the work of the antibiotics.

I took my final capsule on Easter Monday and told my two sons what had been going on. I also let a couple of friends know.

Two days later, as the urinary upsets cleared, I was suddenly poleaxed by a horrible, persistent pain in my right side, which eased off a little as my son drove us to watch a Luton Town game, and continued easing during the disappointing 2-2 draw. But once home I went straight to bed, only to awake at about 2am to get up for a trip to the bathroom, and for the right-side pain to kick in again as I tried to return to my slumbers. I slept only sporadically and at one point very nearly asked Sheila to call an ambulance.

Fortunately, when I then woke again at 6am the pain was gone. I had a GP appointment a day or two later and she told me she thought the right-sided pain could have been down to a kidney stone – another concern with San Francisco imminently on the agenda. I double checked what I was and wasn't covered for under my travel insurance policy, and unless I paid a substantial supplement they weren't going to cover me for anything remotely connected with PC, so I had to shell out an extra couple of hundred pounds.

On Sunday, 28 April I drove to The Horn pub in St Albans, where I had arranged to meet Mount V-, PC-chum Ron at a record fair. I bought LPs by Ten Years After, and West, Bruce & Laing, while Ron snapped up a Moody Blues LP and a couple of others. Then we stood in the bar and had a drink – tomato juice for me, Diet Coke for Ron – and chatted about our recent experiences, gorily comparing notes and trying to convince each other it had all been a piece of proverbial, knowing full well that it hadn't for either of us.

Ron was still coping with frequent 'bathroom stops', and told me he'd only just heard about pelvic floor exercises – which I'd been working on for some time, with some success. We agreed that mentally accepting and coming to terms with the diagnosis we had each received, almost as soon as they were handed out, had been a positive for us, as we'd both made a decision to ask, 'Okay, so what now, then?' and to get on with the answer without complaining. We agreed that this should not be a one-off meet up and arranged the next for a Friday in the imminent future, when we could share a trip to Hitchin's record shops and markets.

When I arrived home, I realised I'd gone three hours-plus without needing to go. Encouraging.

The next day was Sheila's birthday and I took my brilliantly supportive wife out for the day to Kew Gardens. We had a great time, wandering through the beautiful grounds, looking at the plants sitting by the water, just chilling – not normally my thing.

But I enjoyed climbing the 253 steps of the pagoda, while Sheila made it to the 4th floor before crying *enough*. Then we marvelled at the spectacular tail feather display of a peacock, and strolled back for lunch in a pleasant little café, where I realised my new £650 crown still felt like an intruder in my mouth.

I read an interesting story in the *Daily Mail* the following day, suggesting Mount V had been involved in research which could result in just one, much longer, 'less intrusive' session of radiotherapy, rather than the current multiple sessions.

I had an 8 May appointment for a radiography catch up at midday, and was by now feeling much more confident about being away from toilet facilities for any length of time.

***

'Genetic testing help for patients with most deadly prostate cancer' declared a *Times* story today, 7 May. I couldn't help but think that the frequent stories of this nature, and similar – about upcoming treatment breakthroughs – were usually full of ifs, buts and maybes. I wondered, do those writing them ever wonder how frustrating it is for someone undergoing today's state-of-the-art treatment to read these 'breakthrough' stories – being taunted by how much better off they'd have been if they'd only waited a little longer before 'catching' PC?

In this one, Chris Smyth, health editor of the *Times*, reported that a new gene test for PC patients might identify those who were three times more likely to die early. He quoted Professor Paul Workman, chief executive of the Institute of Cancer Research, where the research was carried out on 429 men, as saying: 'This exciting study has identified which features of advanced prostate tumours are the most important for treatment and survival, and has picked out one gene mutation in particular which has an especially serious adverse impact on how long patients live.' This kind of information could result in those at higher risk receiving more aggressive or targeted treatment.

Two weeks later I was reading that a study of 627 prostate cancer patients who had received treatment, reportedly showed that those subsequently using online follow-ups 'rated their psychological wellbeing and quality of life as better than those having to visit hospitals' – and that the online treatment was cheaper per patient by £38.

However, so far there were only five hospitals with online systems allowing patients to raise problems with a care coordinator, while their PSA tests were conducted via their GP surgery. Men in these systems apparently had ten 'unmet care needs' after eight months, compared with 11 for those on standard treatment.

Clinical Professor in Cancer Nursing and End of Life Care Alison Richardson, of the University of Southampton, told the *Times*, 'If implemented properly, this model gives men back control over their own follow-up while ensuring they can still access the support and care they need.'

***

My radiography review seemed to go okay, and consisted mainly of me complaining about the difficulty of getting antibiotics to fight my urinary infection and my female reviewer being very surprised that my oncologist was to see me the next Monday:

'She usually likes to wait three months before seeing her radiotherapy patients,' she told me.

I wasn't quite sure what to make of that.

18

IN WHICH I HAVE BALL-ACHE

MY LONG-TIME friends, John and Jacqui, who had emigrated to Australia many years ago, had just been over on their holidays and it had been good to catch up with them – it had also saved the cost of having to write them a letter to tell them how I was... That'd defray the £240 I'd had to pay for PC-cover when we went to San Francisco.

It was Monday, 13 May. A gloriously sunny and warm day, which I took as a positive omen as I headed for Northwick Park Hospital for my appointment with Dr A, catching the H14 bus which got me there at just after 3pm. This, the hospital's automatic check-in system sternly informed me, was 'too early' to book myself in, so I sat myself down. A man arrived and sat next to me, clearly mistaking the hospital waiting area for a fast-food café of some kind, as he started to tuck into a liberally garnished sandwich, accessorising it with a packet of crunchy crisps and slurping it all down with the assistance of a bottle of Lucozade. Gourmet time, clearly.

A tiny girl of about two wandered around happily enough, despite her right arm being encased in a cast. Another patient close at hand also began to stuff his face – I'd had my own roast-beef-sandwich-with-Branston-pickle lunch at home.

The machine finally permitted me to check in at 3.17, although I was sure I detected a disapproving look from the screen as it reluctantly told me where to go and wait – the Main Outpatients' Clinic No. 4. The good (-ish) additional news was that the whiteboard showed that Dr A herself was holding court today, from Room 10. Just as I noticed this, she popped her head out of the doorway to talk to a patient.

There were only a few people in the waiting room area, but then I was early. I'd have backed myself to be the youngest male of the assembled septet. Only hushed voices were being utilised in our area, but we were cheek by jowl with Clinic 2 and its clientele seemed of a, shall we say, brasher disposition, and there were rather more of them, too.

I spotted a notice on the wall – 'Live well, with and beyond cancer' ...ooookaay, not quite sure about that. There's also a warning notice – 'Be patient. Patients may have to wait longer than their appointed time. The doctor may require longer than normal with a patient... it could be you!' What, was this some kind of National Lottery parody message?! I examined instead the two large paintings of colourful butterflies on the wall, but failed to see their relevance.

At 3.35 Dr A emerged from her room and strode away from Clinic 4. She was tall, wearing skinny jeans and sporting high-ish heels. Not, one would imagine, your typical oncologist. I could have been wrong, though, as she was the only oncologist I knew. I could see she was now chatting to a predominantly blue-clad, smaller nurse, who was going in and out of the room next door.

Dr A reappeared shortly after and called a name other than mine, which produced no immediate reaction... She waited, expectantly, and a man close by told her: 'They went down there,' gesturing vaguely to some indeterminate area. Only for Dr A to point past him, at an aged gent with a stick slowly approaching in our direction. 'There he is, coming to me...' she confirmed.

The aged one soon arrived at our side, clutching a piece of paper. He was possibly being sent off for a blood test. He was obviously hard of hearing as we were then able to hear almost everything Dr A was saying to him from behind the closed door.

I think I heard the depressing phrase 'Half an hour behind' coming from the mouth of our receptionist, directed at a colleague. It was now nearly 4pm and I was scheduled for 4.15. I was called in at 4.44, but to see a different medic – Dr A's right-hand colleague, I suspected.

I was a little phased that she didn't seem to know that I had finished my radiotherapy and that I'd had an infection – doesn't the right-hand talk to the left, I wondered? She thought that the fact I had only just finished treatment and also suffered an infection meant that I should wait about six weeks to have a blood test, which would be more meaningful by then. She gave me a letter to take along to a different counter where they would arrange for a communication to be sent advising me of the date of my next appointment, at which point I should come up for a blood test a couple of days earlier than that date.

She asked about how I'd found the radiotherapy and asked what, if any, bowel movement or urination problems I'd experienced, and told me I would have to complete at least two years of HRT injections. I was out of there in under ten minutes, feeling it had been a somewhat anti-climactic occurrence.

Anti-climactic was perhaps an appropriate description of the conversation I had – listened to, really – with Nurse Gemma a couple of days later, when I went to have my latest hormone therapy jab. She initially asked me about gardening and erections. I thought initially she wanted to know how I had voted, but no, she hadn't mispronounced 'elections' – well, it was only 8.30am and I wasn't really expecting that subject to, er, come up. 'There's plenty of assistance we can provide,' she told me, taking a step or two of a run-in before administering an expert jab. I did appreciate her frankness and lack of self-consciousness, but it was probably a little too early for me to have such matters on my mind at that stage of my recovery. The jab site was tender for a day or so, but I had no worse effects.

A visit to my dentist seemed to have improved the comfort of my crown somewhat, but it was a surprise to receive an appointment invitation for an ultrasound urinary scan for the day after we returned from San Francisco. Slightly more of a surprise to learn it had been booked for me following my overnight pain a couple of weeks back which, to be fair, I'd pretty much forgotten. Nice to know that someone was taking me seriously.

On 28 May, with only a slight sense of foreboding, Sheila and I flew to San Francisco. On the same day the *Times* reported that Sir Michael Parkinson, now 84, had PC diagnosed in 2013, and that he was 'given the all clear' two years later.

The flight revealed a change in habit, which may have been, at least psychologically, related to PC. For years I've had considerable difficulty in being able to urinate in airborne facilities, but suddenly this didn't seem to be a problem.

Seeing the sheer quantity of upfront TV ads about medication for all manner of illnesses and conditions was a feature of the holiday – including 'the only treatment for "prostate problems" which actually works'. Sheila's long-standing ambition to visit Alcatraz was realised in style, after half a dozen of us were taken on a motorised trip around the city in the company of couples from Alabama and Melbourne. It was a thoroughly enjoyable day, ending with an excellent meal at the McCormick & Kuleto restaurant in Ghirardelli Square, across the road from our hotel.

We flew home in early June, fully refreshed and re-energised, and a few hours after arrival I was on an H14 bus on my way to Northwick Park Hospital for my ultrasound scan, having drunk a litre of water. 'DO NOT', ordered the letter I'd received for the appointment, 'empty your bladder until after the examination is finished. It is very important that you have a full bladder – i.e. you should feel the need to pass urine' – and I certainly did! I had flashbacks to Mount V during the ultrasound, shortly after which, I was relieved (sorry) to hear, that the scan resulted in an 'all normal' verdict which encouraged me to go out for a run. Albeit four days later.

Shortly after I found myself bumping into a long-standing, but 'non-intimate' friend. We asked each other 'How are you?', both answering in a way that indicated 'not that good', but without either of us being remotely specific enough to give the other any idea what ailed him... Men, huh!

I no longer remember the incident, but I notice from my diary that on 19 June I wrote: 'Watching TV, I shifted in my chair and felt a little "pull" on one of my balls. Once I would have paid such a thing no attention. As it was, I was still thinking and wondering about it and what might have caused it by the time I went to bed.'

I still had a bit of 'ball-ache' the next morning, notes my diary, but 'it seemed to ease off'. The next day, 21 June, the indelicate diary detail records that 'my farts are beginning to exude a major stink'.

I'd found a few PC references in the papers during early- to mid-June.

On 3 June: 'Prostate cancer cells blitzed with search-and-destroy radiotherapy' declared a *Times'* headline, over a story penned by Chris Smyth, health editor, which claimed that the method 'targets cancer cells with a nuclear payload' and would kill tumour cells while avoiding side effects.

The *Telegraph* ran the story on its front page, writing that the technique involved is called prostate-specific membrane antigen – or PSMA. Australian oncologist Arun Azad called it 'potentially game changing'. An Aussie study of 50 men had shown an extended survival from nine to 13-plus months, with one in five still alive almost three years later.

However, the technique was only 'offered privately in the UK'. 'It involves up to six treatments, every six to eight weeks, costing around £12,000 each.'

On 5 June 2019... Highlighting its '20-year campaign to raise PC awareness', the *Daily Mail* leader article column noted: 'Groundbreaking work by British scientists has led to a major breakthrough. By personalising medication to a patient's generic make-up, doctors can extend their lives – sometimes by years.'

10 June 2019... Hundreds of UK men are trialling a new screening system for PC, which may eventually be offered routinely on the NHS.

13 June 2019... A team of American doctors have developed a method of detecting tumours in PC patients via a procedure including a biopsy guided by magnetic resonance imaging (MRI) which can be used alongside traditional ultrasound imaging methods. A three-year study showed combining both methods led to the detection of up to a third more cancers.

19 June, and a *Mail on Sunday* feature looked at new drugs which held out hope of improving the treatment for advanced PC. 'Impressive results' were claimed for apalutamide aka Erleada, and enzalutamide, aka Xtandi (available on the NHS despite costing some £3,000 per month) – both of which are 'androgen receptor antagonists'.

On 23 June 2019 I saw Gyles Brandreth performing a one-man show at Harrow Arts Centre – and very entertaining he was, too. During his performance he mentioned that he was wearing 'Tena pants' because of a 'prostate problem', and declared that he was the 'new voiceover' for the product 'on ITV3 in the afternoon' and when he had finished and audience members were filing out, the soundtrack of that advert was played via the in-house sound system.

Brandreth, I discovered, interviewed a high-profile PC sufferer, Archbishop Desmond Tutu in Easter 2001:

And he has prostate cancer. I am told that this could be his last interview, that I will find him frail and easy to tire. In fact, as he potters round his kitchen fixing me a fruit juice, he looks remarkably robust. He is 5'5" but sturdy and clearly full of beans. 'I've been having cryosurgery to zap the cancer,' he explains. 'They freeze the prostate, and zap it.' Another paroxysm of laughter. 'They don't freeze everything around there, man. I want to celebrate my golden wedding in style!'

Desmond Tutu will be 70 in October (2001).

Mention of Tutu's height might seem irrelevant in the context of his illness, but an article in the *Telegraph* I'd discovered from

13 July 2017 had suggested that: 'Tall men are more likely than shorter counterparts to die from prostate cancer' according to 'new research' from Oxford University. At last, a reason to be happy about my less-than-towering height.

On 28 June I drove to St Albans to meet up with Ron. We went off on an excellent record hunt in Hitchin, where we visited three market stalls dedicated to vinyl as well as a couple of charity shops. We both found some new old vinyl to chew over – Ron was very proud of acquiring a '78', and an LP by The Spotnicks, amongst others, while I snapped up LPs by Splinter, Steve Howe, Captain Beefheart and obscure '60s US group, Fox – along with the beautiful cheese and pickle sandwiches Ron's wife Jan had laid on for us.

I was able to tell Ron that I had booked a PSA test for the next Monday, to be followed by an 8 July oncologist appointment. A couple of my recent blood tests had been complicated by collapsed veins, but Monday's wielder of the needle made short work of the task.

The next day, I received a reassuring text to tell me that my PSA level was 'reassuringly low at 0.1'. Brilliant. However, inevitably there was a small 'but': 'The white cell count was a little low – this may just be a post-treatment effect, but worth re-checking in a few weeks.' A couple of days later I'm told nothing needs doing on the white cell front.

Some newspaper stories about prostate cancer are enlightening, bringing one up to date with ongoing improvements to treatment, raising one's hopes that inventive and useful research is taking place... and then there are the stories like the one I spotted on 2 July 2019, in the *Times*, of all papers. If only I'd realised how easily I could have improved my chances of not getting PC! I thought, as I read the story which offered 'Three ways to improve prostate health':

1. Eat cooked tomatoes, drink green tea and espresso
2. Lose fat on your stomach and thighs
3. Run, cycle or row for two and a half hours a week.

Call me a cynic, but: yeah, *right...*

***

For a change one weekend, it was me taking someone else to hospital – Sheila was having an MRI scan at Northwick Park. It all seemed to go well. I was surprised at how different it felt to not be the one preparing for treatment. It did, though, remind me of my own MRI scan, which had involved having a canula inserted, via which to pump something into me... No idea what, of course.

Realised I had no idea what MRI stands for... I still don't. Sheila got up to ask the receptionist, 'Do I need to remove my bra, as it has a metal fastener?'

'Let me check for you... Er, no, yours is a head scan, so no, but if it had been for spine, then you would...'

A shortish man, wearing scrubs, appears at the door – 'Mrs Sheila Sharpe?'

She's off and running at 11.09 and back at 11.37, neither shaken nor stirred – 'No problems, although I desperately wanted to scratch my nose halfway through, but couldn't...'

A day later, Monday, 8 July, I bustled into Northwick Park Hospital, past a man in a wheelchair, sitting and smoking under a large poster requesting people to refrain from doing just that.

On my way to check-in, I was passed by Dr A, striding along, but heading in the opposite direction. I arrived in Clinic 4 at 3.43pm for my scheduled 4.15 appointment. Clinic 4 was packed. Some people were standing, but I managed to find a seat, albeit facing away from the reception desk, and sitting opposite a smart-looking dude with low-slung Chelsea-shoes/boots, but seemingly no socks, double-denim jacket and jeans combo, black T-shirt, dreads and a black trilby. He had in his hands a crumpled appointment letter and envelope. I was reckoning an hour and a half wait, but, hey, I had nothing better to do.

Dr A reappeared. 'I wonder if she's been for something to eat?' said one patient.

'She's nice, though,' noted another, and I agreed, albeit silently.

Then, over in Clinic 5 a gentleman, who just might have enjoyed a recent libation, stood up and declared: 'Jesus, come into my heart and save me from my sins.'

He got a round of applause, which encouraged him to tell us all he'd come in for 'a 50-50 operation' – which he fully expected to survive. Power of positive thinking in action, there. He then decided to come over amongst us in Clinic 4, revealing 'I feel more connected to the people here.' He began what turned into a lengthy diatribe, including the information that 'many come in for a minor thing... [he coughed] ...and they end up in the morgue – they're dead!'

His phone rang, whereupon a member of his captive audience suggested: 'Your God is calling you from on high.'

It was now 3.56 and Dr A re-emerged from her office, talking into her phone, and walked off, returning barely a minute later. 'Daniel Murray' came the call from Clinic 5's receptionist, and as our cabaret recognised his name, he began a lap of honour, shaking hands with all of us waiting in 4 – me last. Then he finally rambled off to be seen. It was 4.12.

At 4.20, Dr A called in her 3.30 appointment.

Someone observed that he had heard on the radio today how many days there were left until Christmas, although he'd forgotten the precise number...

'I think I'll go to a beach somewhere this year,' remarked someone else, but another shut down this possible conversation.

'I don't do Christmas since the wife died.'

Daniel Murray re-emerged and began an encore, waving and calling 'Goodbye' to his captive audience. Dr A called me in at 5.05.

'Sit down, please, Mr Sharpe.' She looked through my notes.

Short, sweet, to the point, she told me: '0.1. Perfect. You'll need to carry on with the injections until next July. How are you coping with them?'

I told her my usual line about getting plenty of sympathy from my wife for the hot flushes... But Dr A got to the punchline before me:

'– NOT!' she smiled. 'I'll see you in six months, take this form to reception.'

I raced to reception. No one was there. I stood there looking useless, wondering whether they'd all knocked off for the day. But a medical lady came over – 'Do you want to hand that in? I'll take care of it for you.'

'Thanks,' I said and walked off out of the hospital with a jaunty air, past, this time, a woman sitting under the 'We request you not to smoke' poster, puffing vigorously away. I looked at her, perplexed, but walked away – for at least six months, I hoped.

It was odd to receive this news. I didn't feel ecstatic, as I supposed I somehow expected it after my GP, Dr K had initially tipped me off about my PSA result. But, of course, I was pleased to hear it from Dr A herself – and her genuine-looking smile was a welcome glimpse of humanity between two people, rather than a professional but run-of-the-mill message to a virtually unknown patient. Nor, of course, did this development mean that I was 'cured'. I told my son, Paul, and Sheila my news when I arrived home. She was delighted and hugged and kissed me. Paul and I shook hands. When I later told a friend whose wife had died of cancer a couple of years previously, he told me how 'terrible, absolutely awful' her oncologist had been.

At lunchtime the next day I eagerly awaited my regular dose of *Doctors* – my favourite afternoon soap. Today's episode was about two male patients with leukaemia, one in his early 50s, the other a teenager. They had been having experimental cell therapy, from the results of which the medics hoped to enhance future treatments. But these two guinea-pig patients – the older one called Graham – both died.

***

16 July 2019... 'Can the prostate treatment tamsulosin make you feel lightheaded?' A *Times* reader asked the paper's Dr Mark Porter, adding, 'I have noticed that my head feels swimmy when I stand up.' Dr Porter responded: 'Feeling dizzy is one of the side effects listed in the leaflet that came with your tablets...' (Hmm, bit of a clue there, you'd have thought...)

27 July 2019... A new blood test, called the Mitomic Prostate Test, can flag up cancer with an accuracy of 92%, and will become available through private healthcare clinics, costing from £450, revealed the *Mail on Sunday.*

Not everyone was convinced by claims for the new test. 'There is still a chance that, used alone, it could give a false positive, meaning a man would still have to have a procedure to discover he didn't have cancer after all... ...more research is needed,' said well-named urologist, Marc Lucky.

19

IN WHICH I AM BRUISED BY NURSE GEMMA'S BLOODY DESTRUCTION

YOU MIGHT think that being signed off by your oncologist would be the end of your worries... but when I contacted my travel insurance providers to tell them the good news, they congratulated me – before telling me they'd be charging an additional £358 to cover me for our next trip abroad, which was to be to New Zealand to see our elder son, his wife and our granddaughter in August 2019. Thanks, PC, that's about a grand you've already cost me in additional travel insurance costs.

We'd just returned from some time in Jersey, which we love, but where I'd suffered from a few stomach and bowel-related incidents. I had also decided that radiotherapy had changed my palate. Meat dishes, in particular, were now generally absent from my personal menu. It was time for my next Zoladex implant (as I had now learned was the correct terminology) – which turned out to be a bloody one...

'Sorry about that,' said Nurse Gemma, 'you'll have a bruise.' She then told me she's leaving the practice.

'No wonder you were a little gung-ho with the needle, then...'

Within days we were wide awake in Petone, just outside New Zealand's capital, Wellington, still wrestling with the effects of jet lag, but very excited at seeing our soon-to-be three-year-old granddaughter, Georgia.

I was reading *The Sunday Star-Times*, a Kiwi newspaper, which featured a full-page advertisement launching a 'Blue September' campaign, with a big 'Go Blue for Our Boys' heading alongside a photograph of a half-dressed man wearing jacket, shirt and blue tie, but on his bottom half – only blue boxer shorts and blue socks.

Blue September is the Prostate Cancer Foundation NZ's (hereafter PCF) annual awareness and fundraising campaign.

'Join me in the fight against prostate cancer' pleaded the ad, explaining that the disease 'kills over 600 men each year' in the country, while 'eight men are diagnosed with this terrible disease every day in New Zealand'. The figures also show that some 3,000 New Zealander men are diagnosed annually with the disease – a number which has been heading upwards in recent years. A story in the same paper said that an amazing 90 per cent of those quizzed, in a survey of more than 500 PC survivors, said it was 'helpful when making a decision (about treatment) to speak with others who had treatment'.

Still in Kiwiland for our 45th wedding anniversary in late August, I spotted an item on Australian TV about an Aussie Rules match being played to raise awareness of PC, between two teams of former star players.

A few days later I was concerned by my ongoing inability to enjoy food and drink, which had never previously been a problem. I was, by now, wondering – even worrying – that the change might be permanent. I'd hate having to admit that I was becoming any kind of vegetarian, having always dismissed it as even a remote possibility!

When I'd returned home, I checked out the website for the 2020 Blue September and it was encouraging people to hold blue-themed events to raise money for the PCF, which receives no government funding and explained:

With one in eight men getting prostate cancer, early diagnosis and effective treatment saves lives. Early detection is key and don't wait for symptoms, many men don't have them when they are first diagnosed. Typically men don't know how dangerous this disease is, they don't talk to their doctor about it, their doctor doesn't talk to them about it, or they simply don't know they may have it as they have no symptoms and don't feel unwell.

***

In September 2019 it was reported by *The Mirror* that 'prostate cancer patients could be cured in as little as a week with new high-dose targeted radiotherapy'. Fantastic, I thought, if true... but lower down in the story, there was a warning that:

The study split 850 patients into three groups given different radiotherapy doses. Three months after treatment, side effects for those on Stereotactic Body Radiation Therapy, which delivers precise, very intense doses of radiation to cancer cells, hopefully minimising damage to healthy tissue, were no worse than for standard treatment. They will be monitored for several years to find if they are truly cured. If continuing trials show humans can tolerate such high doses of radiation then SBRT could be offered on the NHS.

Hmm... The odd ifs and buts were there, then...

11 September 2019... A study published in the *Journal of Urology* forecast that a test which diagnosed over 90 per cent of men with aggressive PC during a trial, could become available on the NHS within five years, avoiding thousands of men having to undergo potentially painful and unnecessary biopsies, risking bleeding and infection. The new test, in tandem with a PSA test, correctly identified 86% of those with PC, rising to almost 93% when 12 genes linked to PC were also searched for.

Two days later: 'Hospitals are meant to start care within 62 days of an urgent referral (for cancer treatment) by a GP in 85% of cases. A recent study showed that nearly three quarters of services in England failed to meet that target, compared with 36% five years ago.' – *The Times* leading article.

The same article quoted Cancer Research UK's estimate that 'by 2027 the NHS in England will need 1,700 more radiologists and 2,000 extra therapeutic radiographers'. It also reported that 'Japan has 107.2 CT scanners per million population. Britain has 9.5'.

In late September, I was idly watching the second series of the quirky *Idiot Abroad 2* TV show in which Ricky Gervais and Stephen Merchant send the lachrymose Karl Pilkington to do various unlikely challenges on their behalf. Today he'd been packed off to see a urologist at St Barts for a 'rectal examination'. Karl wasn't nuts about the idea. He really didn't want to undergo it. However, his tormentors insisted, and he reluctantly disappeared into a private room, reassured by the medic that 'every day of my working life it's what I do. Ten to 20 a day. With the index finger.'

'Do you wear gloves?' enquired Karl.

'Bend your knees up. Take a deep breath. Relax...'

'JESUS! F***ing hell... you're touching a lung!'

'Your prostate's fine.'

'You ARE a doctor, aren't you...?'

'In a landmark trial, Olaparib, one of a new wave of drugs that target specific weaknesses in a patient's tumour, held the disease [prostate cancer] at bay for more than twice as long as existing drugs,' reported Fiona MacRae in the *Times* on 1 October 2019.

The trial, which 'freezes prostate cancer in its tracks' involved 387 men with advanced PC, half of whom were treated with Olaparib, half with existing drugs, and showed that the disease was held at bay for an average of 7.4 months in those treated by Olaparib, compared with 3.6 in the other men.

Eight days later, a *Daily Mail* headline suggested that 'mushrooms slash risk of prostate cancer'. The story reported that 'researchers found the fungus was particularly beneficial for those over 50 who eat lots of meat and dairy, but little fruit and veg'. Whilst reading this I was wondering whether these mushrooms were to be consumed or manoeuvred into various bodily orifices to perform their healing duties.

This was a Japanese study, published in the International Journal of Cancer, suggesting that those who ate (phew) mushrooms – there was no detail about which type of mushroom – three or more times per week, had a 17 per cent lower risk of developing the disease, compared with those eating them less than once a week (i.e., me!)

**

It was early October and I was walking through Harrow town centre when someone called out to me: 'Graham... ? Graham Sharpe?'

I was looking towards the bright sunlight and couldn't make out who this might be, then I recognised old chum Dave 'Army' Armitage. We used to spend countless hours with a band of other mates, playing football in the park all the way through our teenage years. He had become a removals man and we had utilised his professional services when we moved house. We'd bump into each other regularly at Wealdstone FC matches.

But he'd packed the family business in and I couldn't remember seeing him at football for literally years. I always liked him, though and, I thought, him me.

'How are you, Dave?'

'Well, I've got prostate cancer...'

He was a little behind me in the treatment process and was undergoing chemo. 'I'm due to see my oncologist soon, and I'm pessimistic as everyone I ever see coming out of her room seems to be smiling – so surely by the law of averages, I won't be?'

I did my best to reassure him, but our paths haven't crossed since... I hope they will eventually as I do like old Dave...

I got up at 6.45am to take my car in for its MOT, only for son Paul to look at the calendar and point out that it is not due until NEXT week. I heard from Ron Arnold, whose PSA level had dropped lower at his most recent test, which was great news.

**

A three-page article in the *Mail on Sunday*'s 'Health Wealth & Holidays' section, dated 13 October 2019, began with a lengthy headline: 'There's a prostate cancer cure that can spare a man's sex life. So why won't doctors tell us about it?'

Hmm, I thought. Pleased though I have been that the Zoladex hormone therapy implants which I had been having for the best part of two years had been effective in reducing my PSA levels, there was little doubt that it did, indeed, have a certain impact on the old libido. So, what does Sally Wardle's story reveal? I wondered.

She explained that 64-year-old Paul Sayer discovered he had PC and was offered a choice of treatments – 'My surgeon was strongly in favour of surgery. And the radiotherapist told me radiotherapy was better.' Paul had heard of another treatment – high intensity focused ultrasound, or HIFU. But when he brought the subject up: 'My doctors shut down the conversation.'

Eventually, he was referred by his GP to a HIFU surgeon, and duly had the procedure in July 2018. I made contact with Paul, who told me:

My treatment story is very different to most men who have experienced the prostate cancer journey. I am one of the tiny numbers so far to have received one of the latest minimally invasive treatments, known as focal therapy or focal ablation.

Each year in the UK, about 48,000 men will receive a new diagnosis of prostate cancer, about 12,000 of whom will have low to moderate, treatable prostate cancer. However, right now, they will only be offered the same invasive treatments given to men with advanced cancers. This means that these men are unnecessarily suffering side effects which, although unavoidable in more aggressive cancers, can be avoided in lower-grade diagnoses by opting for less invasive treatments. These side effects can include high levels of urinary incontinence and sexual dysfunction, along with the associated psychological, physical, emotional and relationship collateral damage. These issues change lives and destroy lifestyles.

So, back to me. I was one of those with an intermediate diagnosis, and I too was offered the same menu of aggressive treatments. Like so many others, I could have simply accepted this, but I chose to investigate what my actual available options were. I am glad I did as I came across a team at Imperial College London under one of the foremost urology consultants, Professor Hashim Ahmed. The professor and the team were treating men with two NICE- and NHS-approved focal options known as HIFU and cryotherapy. HIFU basically uses ultrasound to generate finely targeted points of heat to destroy just the cancer cells without harming surrounding cells and organs. Cryotherapy does the same but destroys the cancer cells using freezing gas delivered accurately via very fine needles.

I was best suited to the HIFU option, and so in June 2018, I went into Charing Cross Hospital as a day-stay case, spent about two hours under anaesthetic, left the hospital with a catheter fitted for the next week, then got on with my life. In the weeks following my procedure, I couldn't help wondering how different my life would have been had I just conformed and accepted one of the other options offered. I also thought about the many thousands of men every year who were simply unaware of, or not even told about, these options and the lives they were now experiencing as a result.

About three months later, at my follow-up appointment with Professor Ahmed, I got chatting. He explained the frustration he experienced almost daily trying to promote more complete access to the treatments nationally. Sadly, as we probably all know, the NHS moves in years, not months, on these things, and due to that, so many men were suffering poor outcomes unnecessarily. I was only in the fortunate position I was because I was born stubborn. I simply hadn't been prepared to accept being told how much poorer my life would be post-treatment. At 61 years of age, I could boast that I still didn't have to get up at night to wee, I didn't have urinary issues, and still had what I considered normal sexual function (well, as normal as it can be at 61 anyway). I wanted to make sure I reserved as much of that as I could.

So, I decided to put that stubbornness to good use a second time. I started a campaign to champion the cause for these cutting-edge focal treatments, to accelerate the roll-out as quickly as possible and to as many men as possible. I wanted every man with an early-stage prostate cancer diagnosis to have the choice of a better lifestyle outcome. Having about 15 years' experience of working in the charity sector, creating and delivering campaigns for both large and not-so-large charities, I was well placed to get the ball rolling. That is why in early 2019, I founded a brand new forward-thinking and highly effective charity called Prost8 and was proud to include Professor Ahmed amongst the patrons. Together we could fight for better outcomes for a large proportion of the one in eight men who will suffer the fate of a prostate cancer diagnosis.

The Prost8 charity has one primary driver. Fight the system to get focal therapies rolled out faster and wider in NHS hospitals across the UK. Work began to ready the charity to launch the initial campaign in April 2020, but a particular global pandemic closed down all thoughts of that. So, meanwhile, the charity took on a support role for as many patients as possible from all corners of the country and we channelled them into Imperial College Hospital under Professor Ahmed. He and his team did a fantastic job under the circumstances, with most other hospitals being closed to everything but Covid-19 cases.

But now, at last, I am proudly leading Prost8 towards a new launch date in October 2021 with what has developed into an even bigger and better campaign to be titled 1in8. This is derived from the aforementioned statistic that one in eight men will get that awful prostate cancer diagnosis in their lifetime. The campaign will make probably one of the smallest financial "asks" from a relatively small percentage of the population. It works by asking just one in eight of the 24 million adult males in the UK to donate £1. That gives £3 million, which will allow the charity to buy, donate and deploy six initial focal therapy suites into strategic NHS hospitals, at the cost of about £500,000 each. This will potentially open up availability to thousands of men each year. Hopefully, following that, the government and the NHS will feel duty-bound to continue the job we are starting, but we will keep fighting if not and deploy even more suites.

It could be any man who is next, so that simple £1 investment is the most cost-effective way to ensure that the very best facilities are in place when you need them. Men, it could be you or a loved one next, and ladies, it could be a man in your life. Prostate cancer isn't particular. Dad, grandad, husband, partner, son, cousin, friend, colleague – all are potential targets. Remember, caught early prostate cancer is one of the most treatable cancers, BUT caught too late, it is one of the least. I, and the small band of men who have been fortunate enough to have had focal therapy so far, are living testament to the effectiveness of the work of Professor Ahmed, his team and, of course, Prost8. I hope, therefore, that readers of this vital book understand what we are fighting for and join the battle.'

HIFU has been an option for over a decade now, and more info can be found at The Focal Therapy Clinic's website, where HIFU Focal Therapy is claimed to be the 'single biggest prostate cancer treatment in the last 20 years'. Also see, nice.org.uk which, in September 2021, said: 'Cryotherapy may be performed under general or spinal anaesthesia. A warming catheter is inserted into the urethra... Cryoneedles or probes are inserted into the prostate, under radiological guidance... Argon gas or liquid nitrogen is then circulated through the needles or probes generating very low temperatures and causing the formation of ice around the prostate gland, which destroys the tissue.' NICE also encourages 'further research into Focal Therapy using HIFU for localised prostate cancer'.

An examination by America's Mayo Clinic of 47 studies involving over one million subjects, carried out between 2006 and 2017, apparently suggested that males with a dairy-heavy diet (that'll be me, then!) could be up to 65% more likely to develop PC, revealed the *Times* on 22 October 2019.

Not everyone agreed, though, with professor of nutrition and dietetics at London's King's College, Tom Sanders, opining that the research did 'not justify the strong conclusions', suggesting that 'being overweight or obese' were the only factors probably associated with risk of PC.

He said that the World Cancer Research Fund had conducted 'a far more rigorous review'. Cancer Research UK's Sophia Lowe agreed: 'We don't think the evidence is strong enough to warrant a change in our guidance', while Prostate Cancer UK's website declared: 'Eating or drinking lots of dairy products... might increase your risk. We don't know why this is but it might be because of the calcium.'

***

My next Zoladex jab duly happened on 30 October, this time Nurse Sally, despite moaning about the number of flu jabs she had lined up, chooses the right stuff for me and manages to whack it in to my left side without any significant blood-letting. She tells me I'll be due again on 22 January, but I can't book that far in advance so have to remember to do so a month before my due date.

Early November arrived along with another touch of cystitis. Went to see my doc, who wanted to take a urine sample and also organise my next PSA test.

***

'Men who carry a faulty gene commonly associated with breast and ovarian cancer should be offered regular testing for prostate cancer after the age of 40, experts have said,' reported the *Times* on 6 November 2019, explaining that mutations in the BRCA set of genes are known to increase the risk of cancer, and that 'those with mutations in their BRCA2 genes have almost double the risk' of suffering from PC.

A study led by the Institute of Cancer Research reportedly found, according to stories carried in late November 2019, that PC 'super responders', who had exhausted treatment options, lived up to 22 months after immunotherapy, via pembrolizumab. The study of 258 men indicated that one in 20 men responded to this method.

A PC test using urine samples taken at home could give a much earlier indication of a need for treatment than is currently possible, it was reported in November 2019. Rhys Blakely, science correspondent for the *Times*, wrote: 'The Prostate Urine Risk test analyses activity levels of 35 different genes contained in parcels of genetic material secreted by the prostate to gauge the aggressiveness of a tumour.' The new method could ultimately obviate the need for blood tests and biopsies. Jeremy Clark from the University of East

Anglia's Norwich Medical School, is leading the ongoing research and declared that it could 'really revolutionise diagnosis'.

***

My mind was diverted from worries about cystitis by the official launch in a local bookshop of my latest title – this one all about my love of records, record collecting and record shops – *Vinyl Countdown*. All went well and the shop reported a record (sorry) turnout for an open function and sold every copy of the book they'd had in stock.

On 3 December 2019 I read, in a front-page story, that using ultrasound to treat some forms of PC 'eliminated the disease in almost two thirds of cases with minimal side effects'. This was found in a study presented at the Radiological Society of North America, and the article in the *Times* explained that the procedure involved sending 'precise doses of sound waves to diseased prostate tissue while sparking the healthy nerve tissue' surrounding it.

However, some experts believed that ultrasound was 'unlikely' to be as effective as surgery or radiotherapy in eliminating the disease, but was less invasive and may have fewer side effects. The procedure involves using a rod inserted into the urethra while the patient is inside an MRI scanner.

Prostate Cancer UK's Simon Grieveson commented that it was not clear yet, from the results so far obtained, 'whether this could be as effective as the treatment options currently available and if so which men could benefit the most'.

It was suggested that 'routine screening every four years for men at risk of prostate cancer could prevent one in every six deaths from the disease', according to scientists from University College London, in a *Times* story on 21 December 2019.

***

As Sheila and I saw the New Year in at a favourite local restaurant, Friends, we enjoyed a high-quality meal and some low quality, hugely and discordantly loud bagpiping, which was rather less to my liking. But it was an opportunity to reflect on making it to the end of the year in some sort of positive frame of mind, having survived what could have proved a major life crisis. And if terrible bagpipe music was the worst I would have to deal with during the next 52 or so weeks, then I'd happily listen to several-LPs' worth of the caterwauling.

20

IN WHICH I SUFFER FROM BUSTED CLUTCH

RETURNING FROM an early New Year trip to Christchurch – no, not the Kiwi one – a mere three days into 2020, my previously completely reliable Audi conked out on the motorway with what the friendly and efficient AA man diagnosed as a busted clutch. This left me worse off by a four-figure sum, and hoping this wasn't a mechanical omen that pointed towards biological batterings under my own bonnet to come.

My first medical complaint of the year concerned wrist and shoulder problems which, in hindsight, seem to have been a little wimp-ish to draw to my GP's attention, and certainly not PC-related.

Then Monday, 13 January 2020 saw me heading for my Northwick Park Hospital 4pm appointment. As ever, the waiting-room cabaret was provided by fellow patients, one of whom was waiting for his dad to be seen, but was most exercised that he was unable to 'get my meds' without having to take time off work, but was promising himself 'I'm gonna go and see 'em to sort it out'.

The female member of an elderly couple nearby told her husband: 'Ooh, look at that, four of them have been in to see Dr A.'

'I've got no choice, I'll go and see 'em about my meds this evening,' declared the nearby son.

Dad riposted with: 'They won't let me have the tablets before I see the doc. She's got to be six feet tall and she wears six-inch heels.' At which point Dr A emerged.

Son says, 'Yeah, she's a nice woman.' I was pleased to hear we agreed about that.

I got in to see her about half an hour after the scheduled time, but I was not worried about that, and she didn't seem too worried about me, suggesting that all was currently well but that I should continue with the Zoladex injections until I'd been on them for two years. At this point she'd get me to have a PSA test and then decide whether I needed to continue with neither, both or one of these treatments. This put my mind at rest for the time being.

Three days later on 16 January, an article appeared in the *Daily Mail*: 'Prostate deaths hit record high...' read the headline for the page-10 story, under their 20-year+ campaign banner of 'END THE NEEDLESS PROSTATE DEATHS'. The story revealed that PC deaths had passed 12,000 in a year for the first time, up by 27% over the course of under 20 years, from 9,460 to 12,031 in figures compiled by Prostate Cancer UK. 'By 2030 prostate cancer is set to be the most commonly diagnosed of all cancers in the UK.'

There was, though, also good news, attributed to an NHS spokesman: 'The survival rate for prostate cancer is now at a record high of 86%.'

Record high deaths, AND record high survival rates, though – how can they both be the case, I asked myself? I then told myself, well you see it is because the number of people who get PC has increased, but so has the percentage of the total who survive. Even though the proportion who die, out of those diagnosed, is less, because overall numbers are up, so are deaths. The former is measured by the number of deaths, the latter is measured as a percentage.

I was supposed to be meeting up with cancer pal Ron one Sunday to check out the St Albans Market for vinyl, but with the Hatters playing an early morning kick-off game, which was live on TV, I decided to opt out on this occasion and told him, 'We'll definitely go when the next Market takes place.' But by the time the next scheduled one came along, the world was busy converting itself into coronavirus crisis mode.

As early as Wednesday, 22 January I had my next Zoladex appointment. Nurse Sally told me her father (or father-in-law?), now in his 90s, had been having such jabs for ten years – 'He'll die with it, rather than from it.'

A week later Sheila and I met up with my travel agent friend, Jeff Lockwood, to discuss the question of where I should spend my 70th birthday on 23 November 2020. When I was 50, we'd gone, with friends in tow, to Paphos in Cyprus. It was such a successful week away that we did the same for my 60th and 65th, but I was now wondering whether it might be time to ring the changes, as some of the friends who joined me now lived in Spain, so if we were to choose a venue near them it would guarantee their involvement and save us a couple of hours on the flights.

We decided to ask one of those now living out there to check out the facilities of a couple of hotels Jeff knew of in Estepona. At the same time, I began looking to book flights to New Zealand for this Christmas and New Year so that we could fly over to see our son, his wife and – by then – four-year-old-daughter, Georgia.

The next day I was due to have lunch with a former boss, but he cried off, ill – 'Just as well you're not in China,' I joked, in a reference to the mystery disease which was appearing there. To assuage the disappointment, I booked tickets to see blues guitarist and singer, Robert Cray, at the nearby Alban Arena in May. Later that evening the UK officially left the EU.

***

'If it were the other way around – if a cancer that killed women attracted half the money apportioned to a cancer that killed men – imagine the outcry. Instead, the news is met with a shrug,' wrote NHS psychiatrist, Max Pemberton, after explaining that 'prostate cancer is now the most commonly diagnosed of all cancers', but adding, 'research into breast cancer attracts more than twice as much funding.' He later declared in this slightly controversial *Daily Mail* article of 1 February 2020: 'White, middle-aged men... are considered to be "privileged" and therefore their concerns are often dismissed.'

***

Another plan to visit the St Albans Market with Ron was scuppered when the 16 February event was cancelled because of the forecasted and imminent arrival of 'Storm Dennis'.

***

A new radiotherapy technique could halve side effects after a way of 'curving' beams to target tumours directly was set to be introduced, reported the *Daily Mail* on 17 February 2020. Radiotherapy treatment is 'highly effective' but carries a risk of damaging healthy tissue and organs, but the new method involves 'intensity modulated radiotherapy' which can be shaped around other parts of the body. Radiologists inject the prostate with tiny pieces of gold, which show up on scans, to help with accuracy. Yes, I knew that, of course, having had it done – David Beckham may have gloried in his 'Goldenballs' nickname, but maybe 'Goldenbum' didn't have the same ring to it.

***

During the next week we enjoyed a trip to London with friends Les and Aydee to celebrate the latter's birthday, by seeing David Mitchell starring in the excellent *Upstart Crow* at the Gielgud Theatre.

The next evening, I was back in town meeting up with long-term pals and racing writers, Sean Magee and Jamie Reid, both of whom have their own chequered history of ailments, while the fourth member of our little group was fellow PC sufferer, and also a racing journo, David Ashforth.

My diary entry for Tuesday, 25 February observes: 'No sign of coronavirus clearing up any time soon, although only 13 people with it here.' Two days later it was snowing. The day afterwards it was pouring with rain and our garden was flooded. There were reports of panic-buying in supermarkets. An 'overreaction' declared my diary note.

On Tuesday, 3 March, Boris Johnson informed us that 'up to 80% of the population may get coronavirus', which I felt was something of an unconventional way of deterring panic-buying... My diary wondered: 'Will we all laugh about this come, say, June?'

The supermarkets were definitely becoming busier with people piling their trolleys high. We don't have a freezer so didn't have much capacity to stockpile, but we were beginning to ensure that we had some reserve tins of stuff stashed away. Just in case...

We attended our regular monthly quiz evening on 5 March and the host, Matthew, announced it was to be his last, as he was leaving for a new job elsewhere. Little did we expect it would be our last, full stop. To commemorate the occasion, the eight of us in the quiz-squad agreed to meet for a meal at The Castle pub at Harrow on the Hill the next week.

At this stage, only a couple of hundred people had been diagnosed with coronavirus in the UK, and reportedly only two had died as a result, but alarming predictions of possibly millions of victims were growing. The government were saying don't overreact or panic buy – but then added that you must self-isolate for weeks if you think you have it. But how could you survive for weeks if you hadn't, well, 'panic-bought' as some will say, or 'stockpiled and taken sensible precautions', as others will phrase it?

Footballers were being told not to shake hands before, during or after matches, yet no mention had been made of spitting. Someone on the radio wanted to calm people down – 'When it gets warmer the Covid-19 threat will diminish.' Erm, other countries where it was currently warm or hot still didn't seem to be avoiding infections, though. By Tuesday, 10 March there were noticeable gaps on our local Morrisons' shelves, virtually all sport had been stopped in Italy and the tennis schedule in the USA was being disrupted.

***

'A blood test promising to revolutionise how prostate cancer is monitored, allowing doctors to identify men who require urgent treatment,' wrote the *Times*' science correspondent, Rhys Blakely, on March 10.

'This test [which, said the article, could cost as little as £150] can tell us, for the first time, whether a man is really at risk of aggressive prostate cancer – it's a very powerful tool,' declared Gert Attard of the UCL Cancer Institute.

The non-invasive test 'looks at compounds known as methyl groups, which become attached to certain stretches of DNA and control the activity levels of specific genes.'

***

The media was already behaving responsibly or dismally – make your own mind up – by ramping up fears with Covid scare stories. This was something which I would find difficult to justify all the way through the ongoing situation, and even bearing in mind that I am a life member of the National Union of Journalists. I would often despair at the political tone of so many articles and press conferences. Whatever happened to just asking and reporting the who, what, how, when, where and why of a situation? I'm not interested in the journalist's personal take on a news story.

On 11 March, Sheila and I decided we would go to our pre-booked Bryan Ferry concert at the Royal Albert Hall. We sat cheek by jowl in the restaurant for an enjoyable meal before the show, chatting to a couple who had to rush for the station immediately after the gig was over, to get home to Nottingham, and were a little concerned in case they missed the train, or it was cancelled.

As usual I seemed to be the only person really enjoying the support band's set. Ferry started slowly but really got into his stride during his lengthy performance. We legged it home as quickly as possible after. And at the time of writing – late November 2021 – we had only recently attended our next gig – starring *The Manfreds* and the great *Zoot Money*.

Friday, 13 March appropriately brought with it an increasingly surreal feel to normal life.

We're in Sainsburys early, but they're short of many items, although there were alternatives, so no genuine prospect of being unable to buy essentials. Toilet paper and bottled water were scarce. Note to self, I thought: collect up as many free papers as you can find, they could be useful if the toilet paper shortage becomes lengthy... There was still little media comment about large gatherings and I risked an evening in the pub with a few mates, none of whom appeared overly concerned about what was to come.

Twitter took on a decidedly 'we're all doomed' air over a bizarre weekend, while supermarkets were packed and other countries announced 'lockdowns', whatever that may mean. It was starting to resemble being caught up in a disaster movie, so Ron and I ruled out a Sunday trip to St Albans Market – that day's papers were full of warnings to this 69-year-old that the over-70s (Ron) would almost certainly soon be forcibly quarantined in their homes for weeks on end.

Monday, 16 March saw Boris warn people not to go to pubs,

bars, theatres and restaurants – although he didn't order them to close. He wanted people to work from home and to avoid social contact. Hmm. Tomorrow we were due to meet six friends at a local pub, The Castle, for a meal, at 1pm, always provided it was still open... Which it was, although we seemed to be the only customers when we arrived. (And still were, by the time we had finished.) Some of us dared to shake hands or hug, others not. Ours was the only table occupied in the pub's restaurant. The meal was excellent; the atmosphere truly weird. We didn't rush, I took photos and my son Paul arrived to collect us at 5pm. We all wondered when we'd be at liberty to do this again. Fortunately, we have been able to do so.

The news told us the UK death toll was now at 71. My son, now working from home as office staff were deterred from attending the office, and his nursery teacher girlfriend were told by their travel company that their impending holiday in Jersey was off, as the island had imposed a 14-day quarantine for visitors. I'll spare you the continuing story of most non-PC related coronavirus news, as you will have your own memory of how it goes from this point on...

***

In an early March 2020 article, whose introduction declared PC was being 'predicted to be the UK's most common cancer', the *Times* writer Peta Bee suggested lifestyle changes which 'may reduce' the risk of PC.

Whilst encouraging men to take a PSA test, Peta wrote that 'about 15% of men with prostate cancer have normal PSA levels' and referenced a study co-funded by World Cancer Research and Cancer Research UK in December 2019 which looked at the effect of 22 risk factors and 'revealed exercise to have the most significant impact'. The article also warned that 'if you are black then the likelihood of getting prostate cancer... is double that for other men.'

The piece then considered dietary benefits – 'Nutrients such as selenium – found in Brazil nuts, fish, seafood – and vitamin E – in nuts, seeds, wholegrains – are important for a healthy prostate.'

The regular consumption of mushrooms, as monitored in a Japanese study of 36,000 men aged from 40-79 over some twenty-plus years, had revealed an 8% lower risk of PC for those regularly consuming the fungus – and a 17% lower risk for those doing so three or more times a week. Tomatoes were closely associated with PC prevention, it was advised, while consuming high quantities of dairy foods had been associated with an increased risk.

'High intakes of alcohol and processed meat products should be avoided,' explained Emma Craske, a Prostate Cancer UK specialist nurse. Obesity was also to be avoided and early treatment for PC to be encouraged, concluded the article.

The same day's paper also ran a story saying that the number of NHS trusts which now had access to multi-parametric MRI machines had risen to 75% from 50% three years ago. These offer tests 'thought to be much more effective than biopsies' (Oh, thanks, how come Mount V doesn't seem to have one?! I selfishly thought.) which 'combine three types of scan to produce a highly detailed image of the prostate'. The figures were welcomed by Prostate Cancer UK's Heather Blake who commented: 'Latest figures show a sharp rise in men referred and subsequently diagnosed in England as they become more aware of their risk.'

***

On Thursday, 19 March I wrote to the publisher of this book with four suggestions for the follow up to my recent *Vinyl Countdown* – I made the crazy idea of writing about prostate cancer the 33/1 outsider of the four to be accepted.

Eleven days later, I realised that it was a good job I wasn't still a bookie. My publisher told me he's opting for the PC idea. Gosh, I'd better start researching and writing it, I supposed!

21

IN WHICH COVID REALLY KICKS IN

I WAS beginning to realise that as the coronavirus measures and cases mounted, the NHS was going to be unable to meet its obligations to those suffering from other complaints - almost certainly including PC patients. The Olympics had been postponed. Hairdressers and dentists were closed. Prince Charles had tested positive for Covid... days later so had Boris Johnson, Matt Hancock and their medical guru Chris Whitty - it's like some corny '50s sci-fi movie, only true...

On 2 April the new ritual of coming out to applaud the NHS began - with a decent turnout from our road, including us. The next day I was out walking and went past the local barbers which was 'Closed by Covid' but showed an 'Emergency' mobile number. Go figure!

Boris Johnson was in intensive care on 6 April. I began looking through my extensive albums of photographs of friends and relatives dating back 40 or more years and putting some of them on Facebook to entertain people. The two events were not connected, but I felt I and probably others I knew might be grateful just to take their minds off a situation seemingly spiralling out of control.

I researched the true story about my cousin who was imprisoned for murder many, many years back. I watched the literally lunatic and unbelievable Netflix series *Tiger King* as the world threatened to spin completely off its axis.

I tried to chase up a date for my next oncologist appointment, prompted by a spate of hot flushes - no, no sympathy whatsoever

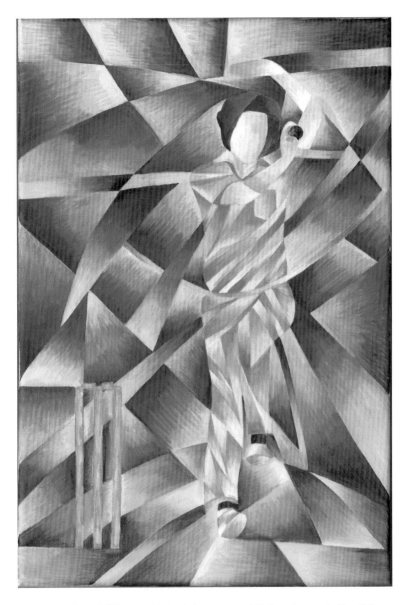

LAUREN'S TRIBUTE... Bob Willis's wife, Lauren, created this instantly recognisable artistic tribute to her cricketing-great husband, whose legendary bowling, combined with team-mate Ian Botham's ferocious batting, double-handedly resulted in a 500/1 come-from-behind England victory over the Aussies in the 1981 Ashes test match at Headingley. Having witnessed his suffering and eventual death from Prostate Cancer, she and Bob's brother David teamed up to form the Bob Willis Fund to raise money to support research into the disease. (bobwillisfund.org)

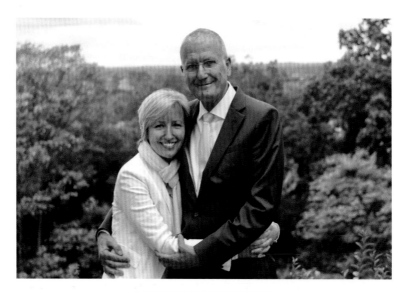

LAUREN CLARK & BOB WILLIS

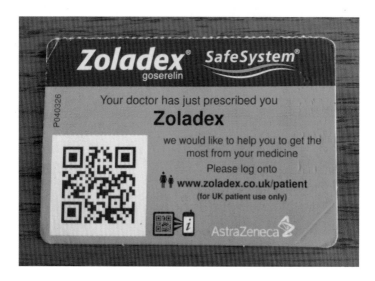

ZOLADEX... 'I knew Zabadak was the title of a Dave Dee, Dozy, Beaky, Mick and Tich hit from the sixties, but I had to learn that Zoladex is the testosterone suppressant which gave my GP practice nurse(s) carte blanche to stab, punch, batter and bleed me every twelve weeks for two years.'

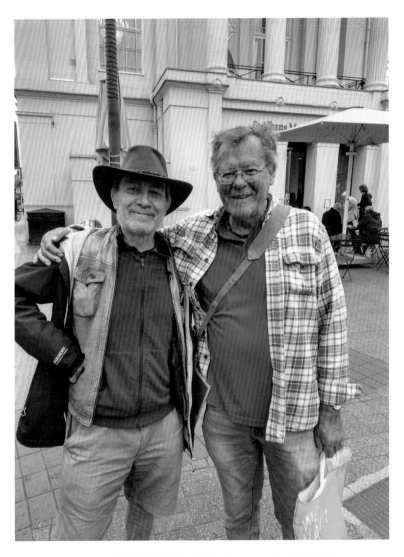

A DAY THEY FEARED MIGHT NEVER COME... Here's the author (left) with his now great mate, Ron, when they met up to ransack St Albans market's vinyl stocks after both completing their Mount Vernon stints, during which they first met, instantly becoming kindred spirits. (Photo by Penny Arnold)

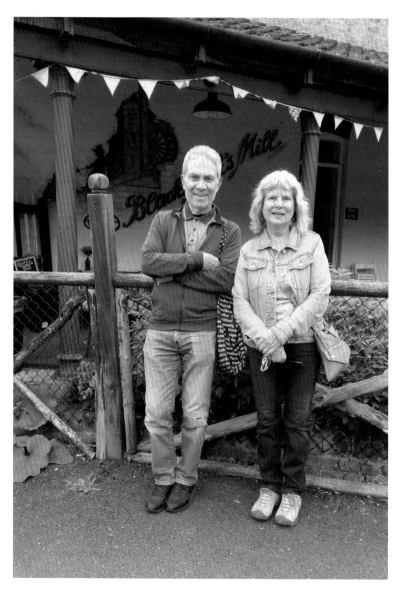

SHE'S THE ONE... Graham's long-suffering wife, Sheila, who took the decision to tell their boys what was going on... married to her for the best part of half a century and convinced he knew her every move, he only found out when he asked her to write a foreword to the book! (Photo by Colin Mason)

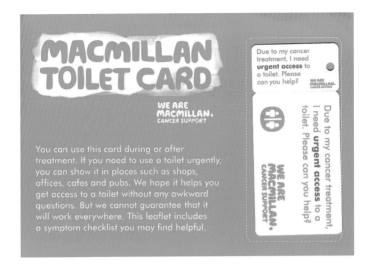

Any PC patient will admit that feeling 'pissed off' is just an everyday occurrence during treatment, but this card offers the opportunity to avoid the ultimate embarrassment which a frequent overwhelming urge to 'go' can threaten.

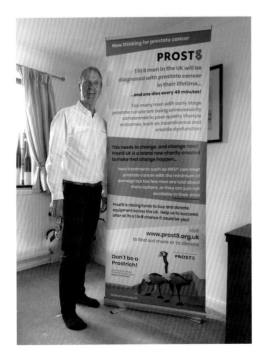

PAUL SAYER was reluctant to accept the guidance he initially received about treatment for his PC symptoms without investigating alternatives. He opted for HIFU, which involves ultrasound generation of points of heat to destroy cancer cells. Impressed by his results he teamed up with a medical professor to launch his charity, Prost8, and its '1in8' campaign aiming to fund focal therapy suites into NHS hospitals. (prost8.org.uk)

Patient Appointment Schedule

Patient ID	First Name		Last Name	Page 1 of 1
444 909 0357	GRAHAM		SHARPE	

Date/Time	Machine			
Feb 4 2019 12:05PM	LA3_2012	LA7	☑	(+ URINE TEST)
Feb 5 2019 12:05PM	LA3_2012	LA7	☑	(+ want to Bring Sham Gr (Am)
Feb 6 2019 12:05PM	LA3_2012	LA10	☑	(Son wary: Lost come up cut off litte)
Feb 7 2019 12:00PM	LA10_2018	LA10	☑	(huge amount myself suit)
Feb 8 2019 12:00PM	LA10_2018	LA 9	☑	(= Amount Shaun Kevin)
Feb 11 2019 12:00PM	LA10_2018	LA 9	☑	k Robin Jumbs.
Feb 12 2019 12:00PM	LA10_2018	LA 10	☑	Pob Fleming
Feb 13 2019 12:00PM	LA10_2018	LA 10	☑	Johnny Wilson
Feb 14 2019 12:00PM	LA10_2018	LA 9	☑	SRC
Feb 15 2019 12:00PM	LA10_2018 LA3		☑	No CD Angel
Feb 18 2019 12:00PM	LA10_2018 LA10	CLINIC	Rad review	
Feb 19 2019 12:00PM	LA10_2018	LA 10	☑	Missy Blues
Feb 20 2019 12:00PM	LA10_2018	LA 10	☑	Robert Cray
Feb 21 2019 12:00PM	LA10_2018	LA 10	☑	Ribs Starks
Feb 22 2019 12:00PM	LA10_2018	LA 10	☑	Bob Dylan
Feb 25 2019 12:00PM	LA10_2018	LA 10	☑	Robin Trower
Feb 26 2019 12:00PM	LA10_2018	LA 10	☑	Hendrix
Feb 27 2019 12:00PM	LA10_2018	LA 10	☑	Cray
Feb 28 2019 12:00PM	LA10_2018	LA 9	☑	Status Quo
Mar 1 2019 12:00PM	LA10_2018	See over →		

Patient Appointment Schedule

Patient ID	First Name	Last Name	Page 1 of 1
444 909 0357	GRAHAM	SHARPE	

Date/Time	Machine		
Feb 27 2019 12:00PM	10 LA10_2018 ✓		Csny
Feb 28 2019 12:00PM	9 LA10_2018 ✓		Status Quo
Mar 1 2019 12:00PM	7 LA10_2018 ✓		Gary Rossini (sorry?)
Mar 4 2019 4:40PM	10 LA10_2018 ✓		Sourthern (Shaun long!)
Mar 5 2019 4:35PM	10 LA10_2018 ✓		PA/GC
Mar 6 2019 2:45PM	20 LA10_2018 ✓		Whiskbone Ash
Mar 7 2019 2:50PM	10 LA10_2018 ✓		Trouble Trunks
Mar 8 2019 2:45PM	10 LA10_2018 ✓ ★ Change name of Room + Moussa Sanctions		
Mar 11 2019 2:50PM	9 LA10_2018 ✓		Linux Johnson
Mar 12 2019 2:50PM	10 LA10_2018 ✓		White Bush
Mar 13 2019 2:45PM	10 LA10_2018 ✓	Clinic Radiographer Review Southern	
Mar 14 2019 2:45PM	10 LA10_2018 ✓		The Who
Mar 15 2019 2:45PM	10 LA10_2018 ✓		Get Around
Mar 18 2019 2:50PM	10 LA10_2018 ✓		Hollies (Carlisi 3 days)
Mar 19 2019 2:50PM	12 LA10_2018 ✓		Free
Mar 20 2019 2:50PM	10 LA10_2018 ✓		Bob Seger
Mar 21 2019 2:50PM	10 LA10_2018 ✓		Status Quo
Mar 22 2019 2:50PM	2 LA10_2018 ✓		Roxy Music
Mar 25 2019 2:50PM	10 LA10_2018 ✓		Kinks
Mar 26 2019 2:50PM	5 LA10_2018		Gene Gunns
Mar 27 2019 2:50PM	9 LA10_2018		Bowie (review)
Mar 28 2019 2:50PM	10 LA10_2018 ✓		Going to stnum!
			(Every thing!)

MY TREATMENT PAPERS… Graham's 'Patient Appointment Schedules' showing his appointment times, changes of venue and intended musical accompaniments. Things didn't always go to schedule as he discovered very early on in the process, although delays helped him to interact with other patients on a daily basis.

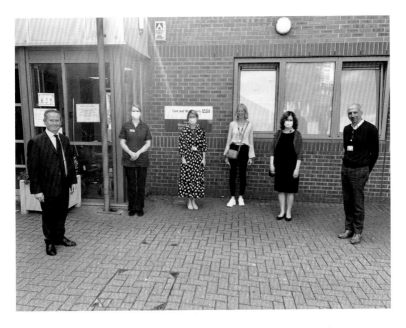

DAVID SIMMONDS, Graham's MP for Ruislip, Northwood and Pinner constituency, has been actively campaigning over the future of Mount Vernon and its cancer facilities.

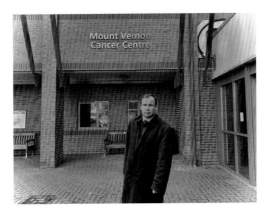

GARETH THOMAS, local MP involved in discussions over the future of Mount Vernon Hospital (gareththomas.org.uk/mount-vernon-campaign/). In March 2021, Gareth made the point that: 'I know many local residents really appreciate the services that are available on the Mount Vernon Hospital site but we need to be honest with ourselves on how this site will function going forward.'

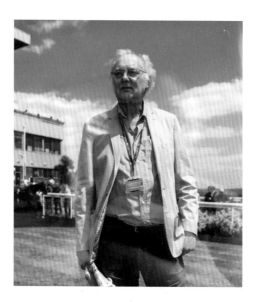

DAVID ASHFORTH, long-serving writer with the *Racing Post* newspaper, who once visited all of the racecourse toilets in the land to determine the one with the best facilities (very useful information for PC-affected racing fans – Market Rasen was deemed the winner, and promptly re-named their ablutions in his honour), tells of his own PC experiences and the advice and guidance he has received from 'Dr Glum'.

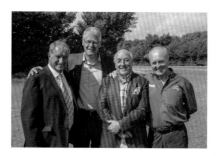

Left to right: **BOB CHAMPION**, Grand National-winning jockey (on Aldaniti in 1981) and founder of the Bob Champion Cancer Trust (bobchampion.org.uk) which supports research into Prostate and other forms of cancer and raises funds for the Bob Champion Cancer Research Laboratory. He was appointed CBE in the 2021 New Year Honours 'for services to prostate and testicular cancer (from which he suffered) research'.; racing journalist and broadcaster, **MIKE CATTERMOLE**, BCCT chairman; with former leading jump jockeys, Champion Hurdle-winning **RICHARD PITMAN**, who also finished second on Crisp in a desperately close finish with winner Red Rum in the 1973 Grand National; and cancer sufferer **JONJO O'NEILL**, who not only won both the Cheltenham Gold Cup and Champion Hurdle twice, but also trained Don't Push It to win the 2010 Grand National.

from my good lady-wife, of course – but didn't get far. Boris seemed to be hanging on in there.

'PROSTATE CANCER RESEARCH IS AT A STANDSTILL' warned a large, third-of-a-page advertisement in the *Metro* on 14 April, placed by Prostate Cancer UK, asking for donations to ensure that 'vital research into better tests and treatments... is not lost due to the impact of Covid-19.' Given the unprecedented situation, I was beginning to rethink my attitude towards the funding of such organisations. At least temporarily.

The next jab day arrived on 15 April. I was to see Nurse Sally and I idly wondered whether she might now, because of social distancing, have to administer much as a darts player might – aiming at me from a distance and hurling the syringe at my stomach.

She pretended to ponder, then: 'Suppose I'd better put on my PPE,' she joked, before swinging straight into action:

'Oh,' she said, sounding surprised, 'No blood.' That cheered both of us up.

Once again, my internal monitoring resulted in the belief that I might yet again have a urinary infection. I managed to contact the GP for a telephone consultation, and was prescribed antibiotics, which I went to collect, and while I was there bought my first anti-Covid masks.

My wife was devastated to receive a phone call from her best friend telling her that she has a very serious, cancer-related condition, which may not have a positive outcome. Sheila was understandably very upset for the rest of the day, as she tried to come to terms with the news.

Having worked for a bookmaking company for 46 years, I tend to look for appropriate names of horses to back as I long ago realised that studying form doesn't appear to equal potentially profitable bets. I spotted a horse called 'Blame Bishop' running on 25 April. A very good mate of mine is called Mike Bishop, so I told him that this must be a horse for him to back given I have blamed him for many things over the years.

He put £3 on it at odds of 22/1. Of course it won, making him a £66 profit. Me? No, I won nothing – I'm not stupid enough to back horses because of their names!

As lockdown shut things down, I decided to try to do the things I'd always said I'd get round to doing. One of which was to try to track down a once very good friend of ours who had married another good friend, but he, the latter, died of cancer in his late 20s, after which we stayed in touch with her for a while but she eventually moved away.

Enlisting the help of other friends via Facebook, Twitter, emails and phone calls, we eventually managed to discover a phone number for her. Plucking up courage I rang the number, which turned out to be for our mislaid friend's daughter by her second husband. However, she had bad news to relay – that her mum had died a couple of years ago, aged 64. This news saddened us all, but at least we knew, and the search did put us in touch with other lost acquaintances who were still around to chat over old times.

The 29 April, was Sheila's first lockdown birthday – we celebrated with a trip to Waitrose, a Skype from granddaughter Georgia and a takeaway from the excellent local Steak restaurant, washed down with champagne.

Following on from an October 2019 story, the *Times* of 29 April 2020 quoted a consultant medical oncologist at the Royal Marsden NHS Foundation Trust as saying that breast cancer drug Olaparib 'which targets an Achilles' heel in cancer cells while sparing normal healthy cells, can outperform targeted hormone treatments in some men with advanced prostate cancer.' They added: 'Next we will be assessing how we can combine Olaparib with other treatments which could help men with prostate cancer live even longer'.

This really did seem to be a promising development.

22

IN WHICH NATURE DECIDES TO DOWNGRADE PC

INSPIRED BY the example of my cancer friend Ron, who could turn his hand to loads of mechanical and practical stuff, I made a real effort and after just some – well, three – hours, I'd managed to change the stylus on my record deck. Exhausted by that supreme effort, I sat down to read the *Mail on Sunday*, on 24 May 2020, and as I did so I felt a wave of heat enveloping me. Oh, here we go again, I reminded myself, it's a side effect of my Zoladex treatment.

Then I spotted the headline: 'Hormone clue to why virus kills more men.' And began reading the fascinating story which was suggesting that men like myself, on treatment for PC which works by reducing testosterone levels 'should', according to Professor Nick James of London's Institute of Cancer Research (ICR), be 'protected (from coronavirus) relative to men who are not on such treatments – meaning most men'.

The paper's medical editor, Stephen Adams, wrote that 'PC experts have now uncovered intriguing clues that the sex hormone testosterone seems to play a crucial role by inadvertently helping the virus infect cells. Italian doctors had found that patients on such treatment "were four times less likely to die of Covid-19 than those not on them".'

I fanned myself whilst reading this apparently and unexpectedly good news for myself and other PC patients, and silently agreed with Prof James that 'being on these drugs [was] the male equivalent of going through the menopause'.

As we moved from May into June, I read that Professor Paul

Workman of the ICR had greeted the results of a pilot study into whether DNA testing in GP surgeries would be a 'safe and feasible' way of spotting those at risk from PC. The pilot tested 307 men, aged between 55 and 69 and identified PC in a third of apparently healthy men who were found to have the highest levels of inherited risk. A larger study of some 5,000 men was planned as a follow-up.

A day later, Prostate Cancer UK reported that 'prostate cancer [had] overtaken breast cancer as the most commonly diagnosed form of the disease. The change – with 57,192 prostate cases in 2018 and 57,153 breast cancer cases – was largely due to increased awareness.'

A *Daily Mail* comment column justifiably congratulated itself on the paper's efforts to highlight awareness of prostate cancer over many years: 'Thanks to the *Mail*'s passionate campaigning and other awareness initiatives, men are finally getting over their self-consciousness and coming forward for tests. Previously, as this paper put it, they had been dying of embarrassment. '

On the same day, however, Prostate Cancer UK's chief executive, Angela Culhane, was warning people: 'We know that the Covid-19 pandemic will have knock-on effects on diagnosis and treatment for prostate cancer for some time to come.'

News was also reported that two UK trials – PROSTAGRAM and ReIMAGINE – were looking at whether a 15-minute MRI scan could prove more accurate than the PSA test.

More (for newer PC patients) news, that fewer radiotherapy treatment sessions could become the norm, was carried by the *Daily Mail* on 21 June 2020, suggesting that 'weeks of back-to-back hospital visits' – I had 39 of them with only weekends off – could be reduced to 'five days of treatment, or even less'.

Trials conducted, delivering bigger doses of radiation over fewer sessions, had been proving successful, and not causing additional side effects.

So many of these stories included a 'could' or a 'possibly'. It's wise not to get too excited by them until they became 'definite's.

The government's National Shielding Service, of which I'd never heard, texted me – 'Please expect a call from us on 03333050466 to register any needs around food, care and wellbeing.' Suspecting a scam of some kind, I had completely ignored, and effectively forgotten about it until an unexpected letter arrived.

'We understand that your GP or hospital specialist has reviewed your medical record and has advised that you are no longer considered to be at the highest risk of severe illness from Coronavirus. This letter is to confirm that the Government is no longer recommending you follow shielding advice.' That's a relief, then, I thought, even though it went on to tell me that I could still ask for help collecting shopping, medicine or other essential supplies that one might need to be delivered to your home. A continuing supply of vinyl records on a regular basis was pretty essential for me, but Sheila told me that she thought the government were unlikely to help with that.

On 27 June, it was reported by the national press that Prostate Cancer UK had called for NICE to reverse a decision denying thousands of men with advanced prostate cancer abiraterone which could cut the risk of them dying within three years by a third, on the grounds that it was not cost-effective. The drug works by blocking the production of testosterone and slowing down cancer growth. Oncologist Dr Danish Mazhar of Cambridge University Hospitals NHS Trust, was quoted as saying: 'Evidence shows that abiraterone has far fewer adverse side effects compared with chemotherapy, and could give these men the additional months of life that they would otherwise miss out on.'

My GP practice sent me this ludicrous text on 30 June 2020 – 'Thinking about your recent appointment – overall, how was your experience of our service? Please reply 1 for Very good; 2 for Good;

3 for Neither good nor poor; 4 for Poor; 5 for Very poor; 6 for Don't know.' On how many levels was this pointless box-ticking of the worst kind? Still, the day before they'd sent me a text explaining how to 'wear and make a cloth face covering'.

Meanwhile, my wife's GP had contacted her, suggesting – sorry, requesting – that she 'have a thermometer, a blood pressure machine and a pulse oximeter at home. These low-cost items can be purchased online or at your local pharmacy. These home devices will help to reduce cross infection and reduce the need to unnecessarily visit the surgery.' In other words: we'd rather you started taking on some of our workload at your own expense.

***

Until I started actively seeking it out, I clearly hadn't realised just how many PC-related stories appeared in the press. The trouble was that those stories, many of which were promising or 'revealing' significant breakthroughs, seldom got followed up. Sometimes, though, they could tell you stuff you didn't know, but perhaps should have done.

On the Bluecrest website (a company offering private health checks), on 1 July 2020, I found this PC-related information:

Men with larger waist circumferences have an increased risk of both developing and dying from the disease. Every 10cm increase in waist size was found to lead to a 13% rise in the likelihood of developing aggressive tumours. Each 10cm increase also leads to an 18% increase in the risk of dying from the disease.

Conversely, men with a healthy body weight were found to have a reduced risk of prostate cancer and death from the cancer. The lead researcher of the study, Dr Aurora Perez-Cornago of Oxford University concluded: 'We need to do further work to understand why the differences in risk exist.'

A BBC Panorama report suggested that 'we may see as many as 35,000 excess cancer deaths as a result of coronavirus' wrote the *Daily Telegraph*'s Allison Pearson on 6 July 2020 – who also, maybe controversially, answered, in her article, the question: 'Why I didn't clap to mark the NHS's birthday' – 'How can it be that minimum-wage supermarket workers manage to greet customers through Perspex screens but highly rewarded doctors couldn't do the same for patients?'

Eight days on, and I read in the *Daily Mail*: 'Prostate cancer has been convincingly linked to the sexually transmitted human papillomavirus (HPV) for the first time.' This is the virus which causes cervical cancer in women. The same article suggested that prostate cancer 'affects more than 57,000 men a year in the UK' and kills 12,000 men in Britain each year.

A further couple of weeks passed, before, on 28 July, a newly introduced treatment – Rezum – for dealing with an enlarged prostate was featured in a *Daily Mail* article. 'Blasts of steam from a device inserted into my urethra would destroy enlarged tissue, removing the blockage which was narrowing the urethra,' explained patient, Simon Dutton, who had the procedure at Hereford County Hospital and was able to return home after four hours. 'Within two weeks everything was working perfectly again. The treatment has given me my life back.' Such treatment reportedly cost the NHS some £2,300 and was available privately for between £3,000 and £5,000.

In early August, the *Mail*'s health editor, Sophie Borland, wrote: 'The NHS is making available more than 50 drugs which can be administered at home, including those for prostate cancer, (enzalutamide and abiraterone which can be taken by men at home instead of having chemotherapy), bowel cancer, leukaemia and a form of blood cancer.' This seemed to contradict recent stories suggesting abiraterone was being denied to patients by the NHS.

Eleven days later, I learned from the *Metro* that: 'The number of patients waiting more than 18 weeks for routine hospital treatment in England has hit a record 1.85m in June as the virus put pressure on services... A total of 153,134 urgent cancer referrals were made by GPs in England in June, down from 194,047 at the same stage of 2014.'

Professor Karel Sikora, an oncologist for 50 years and ex-director of the WHO Cancer Programme, tweeted on 16 August: 'The whole country ground to a halt for Coronavirus, so why is there not more outrage for cancer patients? I've seen a lot in my half century in medicine. I've never been more worried than I am now. This is an unfolding disaster, and so many aren't seeing it.'

In late August I read an intriguing piece, indicating that research produced by Oxford University, in a study involving pooled data from 12 previous European studies covering some 60,000 patients, concluded that doctors are more accurate at diagnosing cancer when they trust their own 'gut feeling' over official symptoms. The research suggested that a patient was over four times as likely to be diagnosed with cancer than when no gut feeling at all was recorded. The more experienced a doctor was, the greater the chances.

Short and to the point, though not the most elegantly phrased, a *Metro* article on 2 September 2020 cut to the chase: 'Men with beer bellies are at increased risk from prostate cancer. The quarter with the biggest waists are 35% more likely to die of it than the trimmest quarter, say Oxford University researchers.' The story did not make it clear whether those with 'wine waists', 'stodgy stomachs', 'quarter-pounder quads' or 'burger bellies' were as equally likely to be at risk.

Mind you, the up-market *Times* also opted to target the same aspect of the story and enlarged the detail – that men with waist circumferences of over 103cm or 40 and a half inches – are 35% more likely to die from PC than the quarter with measurements below 90cm/35 and a half inches. The *Times* added that 'there was no link between body mass index (BMI) scores, which are usually used to diagnose obesity, and prostate cancer deaths' evident from the UK Biobank study, involving 218,225 men who had been followed for over ten years, during which 571 of them had died from PC.

Before I'd read this story, I'd made a visit to my local betting shop - a branch of Coral - where I came away with a flier apparently encouraging me to 'self-exclude from more than one bookmaker in your area' by calling the 'Self-Exclusion Helpline' should my betting habits cause me problems. It made me wonder why every branch of Greggs, or other cake and sandwich outlet, weren't being encouraged to hand out similar leaflets on behalf of PC, warning any men whose stomach diameters were approaching danger level, that they wouldn't be served if they requested too many buns, pasties and cakes? The answer, of course - at least in my opinion - is that this is still to some extent a free country, and just as anyone wanting to gorge on chips, burgers and kebabs was completely at their liberty to do so, so should I be permitted to place whatever bets I wanted in a betting shop without being hectored about my decision!

***

During Covid lockdown it became difficult, nay impossible in my case, to get a haircut. So I decided to let it grow, which it proceeded to do, pretty quickly. I also decided that seeing as longer hair wouldn't really work with the spiky style I'd had for several millennia, I thought I'd reach back in time and comb it into a 'Steve Marriott' style - middle parting, two curtains each flicked over an eye. I thought it worked well. Most people remained tight-lipped when I asked them for an opinion... and some were downright sarcastically rude when I posted a photograph of it on Facebook.

My sister declared that I didn't suit 'flat hair'. Sheila kept her counsel - to humour me, I felt. I never really got the impression that her heart was in it. Anyway, I liked it, so when Karl finally deigned to re-open I dashed over and got him to formalise the style. Possibly against his better instincts... and, soon, against mine. When mid-September came around and the weather was still warm, and I had two floppy flaps of hair protruding into the corners of my eyes, I took the decision to revert back to good old spiky.

After leaving my 'track and trace' details on the counter notepad (old school, I was pleased to note – no instruction to 'use an app', 'send me a text' or any of that nonsense in sight there), I was temperature-zapped and deemed fit to be hair-washed. After one of the best such soapy dowsings I could recall, I was ushered into the cutting chair. Karl assumed I was going to keep it the same but perked up noticeably when I told him that I was reverting back to old faithful, and settled down to snip contentedly away. Until that was, I mentioned the fishing trip he'd just returned from, which I'd learnt of from his colleagues.

He nearly downed tools. Or tool, singular... scissors, that is... and launched into a rant about the woes of an angler, including being stranded in the middle of an unfamiliar stretch of H_2O with no lights to enable him to see where he was. And inflating a newly purchased plastic mattress marked 'Made in China' to sleep on, only to spot a large arachnid of uncertain origin looking at him with malicious intent. When he complained to his friend, who'd organised the trip, saying, 'I didn't see any of this in those photos you showed me,' he was told: 'No, they were of somewhere else.'

Karl reminded me that his daughter was a nurse in the radiotherapy unit at Mount V and then said: 'I had a narrow escape recently when I went to see my GP.'

'Oh yes? How was that?'

'Well, at the end of the appointment she said to me that I was at that age where it might be a good idea for me to have my prostate checked.'

'So, how did it go?'

'I made an excuse and got out of it. I didn't fancy that. And she's a woman.'

'Well, listen to me, Karl. I'm serious.' I told him. 'If you don't have that test done before I come for my next haircut, I'll walk away and go somewhere else...'

***

'Lives at risk in cancer research cash crisis' screamed the 14 September front-page lead headline in the *Daily Express*. It explained: 'Britain's biggest cancer charity could be forced to sack 1,500 scientists because of a Covid funding crisis.' Cancer Research UK was facing having to 'slash research funding by £450 million over three years', having 'already announced cuts of £44 million' that year.

I went to the Cancer Research UK website to check out its current offerings on PC, and was a little surprised to see their PC section had been 'Last reviewed' on 22 May 2019. I knew they probably wouldn't have sufficient staff to be updating it every day, but almost a year and a half since changing the information was not impressive.

On 14 September 2020, I discovered something more positive. Amazon notified me of the following: 'This is your quarterly AmazonSmile donation notification. Your chosen charity, Prostate Cancer UK, recently received a quarterly donation of £3,635.99 from AmazonSmile, thanks to customers shopping at Amazon Smile.' No, I didn't contribute that whole three and a half grand-plus!

The next day, 15 September, the *Express* went back on the attack, once again leading their front page on the scandal: 'Backlog of cancer patients awaiting treatment is "past point of no return". FOR THE SAKE OF 35,000 LIVES... WE MUST ACT NOW.' The story quoted Professor Pat Rice, chair of Action Radiotherapy, and founder of Catch Up With Cancer, saying: 'It's no longer a question of will cancer patients die unnecessarily, but how many will die unnecessarily?'

The paper backed up the severity of the situation by featuring 61-year-old Edinburgh grandfather Keith Roxburgh's experience back in 2012 when he 'was given five years to live' with advanced PC, but after treatment 'here [he was] eight years down the road'. The implication was clear – if he was to present with those symptoms now, he'd be unlikely to get the treatment he desperately needed in time to save him.

Several daily newspapers on 23 September 2020 carried the news that Macmillan Cancer Support was planning to cut 310 jobs, following a predicted fall in its funding of £175m by the end of 2022. 'The coronavirus has had a catastrophic impact on our finances,' explained chief executive, Lynda Thomas.

23

IN WHICH I WHISTLE THROUGH MORE TREATMENT

'IT'S FINE to simply have the next PSA test in six months' time before your next clinic review and proceed with your final Zoladex as planned, in September,' my GP declared in early September 2020.

The next day I had my flu jab, scheduled for – very precisely – 8.51am. I joined the relatively well behaved short queue on arrival, standing behind one of my former Hatch End FC managers, Derek Mowle, and his wife Linda. We were chatting happily when a couple of their (more elderly) friends turned up and began a subtle attempt to insert themselves into the queue in front of us. An equally subtle interchange of body language, opinions and comments ensued in which the three of us made it clear we weren't happy about them doing this. The husband took the hint and moved to the back of the queue while the wife persisted until realising resistance was futile and joining him. A very suburban battle of wills, which could easily have appeared in a 70s sitcom featuring June Whitfield and Terry Scott, or more recently, Richard Wilson and Annette Crosbie.

Some red-looking stools were evident the next morning, and again – albeit a little less so – the one after. Certainly it seemed to feel as though, if I had to strain at all then this would occur, whereas when it was a 'natural' movement it was more, if not completely, normal. When I'd mentioned this increasingly common occurrence to the GP a couple of weeks back, he said he'd make an appointment for me to get some tests, but it could take some time. I thought he had mentioned October...

I read the following in a *Daily Mail* article of 21 September, taken from the book *How To Live* by Professor Robert Thomas: 'We were able to prove that drinking two to three cups of tea a day reduced the prostate cancer risk.' I began wondering: well, why did I get it then? As I'd done that for donkey's years! Then I read on a little, to discover that 'interestingly, there wasn't a benefit for those tea drinkers who added sugar to their cups, however...' I immediately thought – ah, that's why! I've always had something of a sweet tooth, I'm afraid, so have seldom drunk any cups of 'rosie' without the addition of a little of Tate & Lyle's finest. But, as a result of reading this small item, I immediately vowed to no longer have tea in my sugar and banned myself from putting anything other than milk into my morning cuppa. However, I soon began to lapse...

As I wrote this, I seemed to be coping – whilst wondering what blooming difference it was likely to make to my life now – and why didn't the prof, whose research involved 155,000 tea drinkers over a period of 12 years – scribble out his book several – many – years ago so that this information could feasibly have been of any use to me?

Although, I was guessing that as I am also partial to sugar-coated doughnuts and various other sweetmeats containing the substance, it wouldn't have made any difference whatsoever to my chances of contracting PC, and that if it had, I possibly wouldn't have had the pleasure of writing this book...

The same day had also produced a story headlining that: 'Breast cancer drug could transform prostate treatment.' This was the page-4 lead story of the *i* newspaper, giving details of the PROfound trial which was reportedly supporting earlier findings that Olaparib could be successfully used to treat certain types of PC. Researchers at the ICR in London, the Royal Marsden NHS Foundation Trust and Chicago's Northwestern University had concluded that 'the drug should become a new standard treatment for PC.'

Olaparib blocks a protein which helps damaged cells repair themselves, and on which some cancer cells rely to keep their DNA healthy.

A similar article featured in the *Daily Mail* on the same day, about research funded by Prostate Cancer UK, declared that a separate trial had revealed positive news that another new drug – ipatasertib – could result in a 'significant reduction in the risk of the disease worsening or death'. The same paper carried yet another story alleging that the focus on fighting Covid by the NHS had an adverse effect on the extended waiting times cancer patients were experiencing as the attention given to other diseases suffered.

I received another of Ron's uniquely styled emails on 23 September 2020, after I'd sent him one hoping his latest injection appointment would go well. Amongst other news and iffy 'jokes', he wished me 'luck' for what could possibly be my own final Zoladex injection the next week:

Hey mate, thanks for the mail, yep it all went well this morning thanks, hardly felt the needle, whilst Nurse Jackie asked if I would like the shingles jab – apparently it's a one off, lasts forever. I thought that as my hair is a bit thin on top, maybe a few shingles might stop the rain getting in. Whadya reckon? Good luck with your appointment next week mate, let's hope it's the last one. We're off up to see Penny (daughter) again tomorrow – more work, I've made a handrail for their stairs which I have to fix and the newel post at the bottom of the stairs needs re-attaching, and Jan has made cakes and cheese scones, so it's meals on wheels again.

I've got my next jab on the 16 December, that's roughly the same time that the review with the oncologist takes place. I have to wait and see what transpires from that – as you said, it's all a waiting game.

Ron's missives invariably cheered me up – even if I was already feeling cheerful, they added an additional level of cheeriness. I'm so pleased that we have stayed in contact for so long.

In the final week of September 2020, a good friend asked me whether I'd like to come to a 'live' football match on the Saturday afternoon – with real people! Because of the Covid ban on crowds at top-level matches, my season tickets for Championship side Luton Town and National League outfit, Wealdstone – both of which I had been supporting since the late 1950s – weren't actually permitting me to go to the ground to watch a game.

The invitation was to watch the very local team Rayners Lane playing, and I was very minded to attend, until I remembered that on 30 September, just a few days after this match on the 26th, I was due to receive what may possibly be my final Zoladex injection... Now, logically there would have been very little chance of picking up a Covid infection at Rayners Lane, but... but... but... just imagine if I did... I clearly wouldn't have been allowed to attend the GP's surgery for the nurse to administer the jab, which my oncologist had been strongly hinting could be my last if the follow-up PSA test proved to be as encouragingly low as recent ones had been.

Reluctantly, but realistically, I knew I just couldn't take even the tiniest risk that I might pick up some kind of bug at the game, so I decided I should stay at home and watch the horse racing instead. I know, I know. Call me illogical – I was still nipping down to the local Tesco mini supermarket each morning to pick up newspapers and essentials, duly donning a mask once inside and removing it asap when I came out. So what was the logic which would allow me to continue doing that whilst not going to a football match? And I was going out every day for an extended walk with Sheila, where in theory we could come to all kinds of harm. But I knew in my own mind that the 'no-football match' decision was the important one – a random event which wouldn't otherwise even have figured on my agenda at all. This was the gesture that I needed to make to show that I was not being devil-may-care about risks.

I still felt deep down that even if I had got Covid I would have to be hugely unlucky, statistically, to die from it – hadn't my GP already confirmed to me that I was not suffering from any 'underlying health issues'? This was the phrase often used as code by the media etc for suggesting that, yes, this person officially died of Covid (which was not to be encouraged, of course), *but*, after all, they were about to die of something else anyway in the not-too-distant future so, what could they expect!?

Five days later my potential D-day arrived. My 8.30 appointment for my latest and possibly final Zoladex injection from Nurse – rather than Aunt – Sally. I was up bright and early, showered and wearing appropriately loose-fitting clothing to enable easy access to the toned, muscled midriff of which I am so proud... in my dreams! A minor catastrophe as I arrived and pressed the buzzer, after the disembodied voice behind the door responded in Dalek-like tones: 'Do you have a temperature or a cough or a cold? And have you brought a mask with you?'

Feigning astonishment at such questions, despite having dosed myself up the previous night with Lemsip when I'd felt a now absent tickle at the back of my throat, I reached confidently for the mask, which I refused to wear whilst walking along the road, only to notice immediately that one of its elastic attachments had come away... Oh no, they're going to throw me out! I thought. Only for a frantic delving into every possible pocket to reveal another mask – albeit somewhat small for my gob – with securely attached elastic straps, which I quickly donned and then entered the surgery.

A short wait and then there was Nurse Sally welcoming me into her lair and explaining to me that I was her first patient following a two week break. 'You're going to be out of practice, then – perhaps I should come back when you've had chance to ensure that your aim is still true.'

She totally ignored that and motioned me towards the bed, telling me, 'My husband has been made redundant and we're downsizing to a bungalow.'

'Well done for finding one,' I said.

'I narrowed the roads we wanted to live in down to two and made a point of putting notes through the letter boxes of the bungalows I fancied, asking whether they would be thinking of moving shortly,' she said.

Crikey, I was about to be stabbed in the stomach by a bungalow-resident stalker. Good job I live in a semi, I thought.

'Now then which side did I "do" last time?' she mused. 'Ah yes, the right, so...'

'... er, the left, possibly?' I guessed.

'... the left' she confirmed, grabbing a handful of flesh. 'Hmm. Not much to aim at here,' she tutted, at the same moment plunging in the needle/syringe/plunge-y thing, or whichever implement she was using with which to send Zoladex coursing around my system. Always assuming that's how it works...

I mean, for all I still know, it might just sit there and pulse stuff out.

So I decided to check out what had actually been happening to me during these regular injections, and discovered:

The Zoladex implant is inserted through a needle into the skin of your upper stomach, once every 28 days. You will receive the implant in a clinic or doctor's office.

Follow your doctor's instructions. It is very important to receive your Zoladex injections on time each month.

You are not likely to be able to feel the implant through your skin, and it should not cause pain or discomfort. The implant will dissolve in your body over time.

That all sounded accurate enough. Except of course that other than the first couple, my stomach punches had been delivered every three months. I read on and discovered that whether delivered every 28 days or 12 weeks the effects are much the same: 'For the palliative treatment of advanced carcinoma of the prostate: 3.6 mg or 10.8 mg subcutaneously into the upper abdominal wall once. The 3.6 mg dosage may be repeated every 28 days. The 10.8 mg dosage may be repeated every 12 weeks.'

No, I was not going to look up 'subcutaneously' – do it yourself if you're that worried about it!

I also found out that perhaps I should have given up drinking for the duration, as I read:

Avoid drinking alcohol. It can increase your risk of bone loss while you are being treated with Zoladex. Avoid smoking, which can increase your risk of bone loss, stroke, or heart problems. This medicine can pass into body fluids (urine, faeces, vomit). Caregivers should wear rubber gloves while cleaning up a patient's body fluids, handling contaminated trash or laundry or changing diapers. Wash hands before and after removing gloves. Wash soiled clothing and linens separately from other laundry.

Too late, I suppose that's my bones buggered, then... but... 'bone loss'? Really? Where did they go, then? Which ones?!

Once out of the surgery, I realised that I hadn't discussed with Nurse Sally when my next injection, sorry, implant should take place, assuming I had to have another.

After all, although Dr A had told me I may not have to return, she hadn't yet provided me with a date for our next telephone appointment, nor when I should arrange for a PSA test so that she could actually make the decision as to whether I could retire from the implant scene.

Right, so this was intimating that I was indeed imminently going to require some input from my GP in order to co-ordinate competent co-operation, coincidentally, come the next few days.

I set off from the surgery – I had to leave via the back exit, of course, no doubling back on yourself in buildings these days – and almost instantly, having removed my mask, I struck up an involuntary and jaunty whistle. Whistles are always 'jaunty' I believe. I think it may be compulsory for them to be called thus. My long-term hero, (Just) William Brown, pre-teenage star of Richmal Crompton's magnificent series of books, was also an inveterate whistler, of the shrill variety.

Whistling has got me noticed in many situations over the years. Most embarrassingly when I was a regular commuter to London from Harrow-on-the-Hill station where, one morning I was confronted and accused by an attractive twenty-something lady (my own age at the time, I hasten to add!) on the platform who loudly proclaimed, where we were surrounded by commuters: 'You're that whistler!' I could feel myself blushing, as she showed every sign of not wishing to end the one-sided conversation.

I resisted the temptation to retort 'and you're that rarity, a woman who fancies me', and in the time-honoured fashion of fellow journalists over the years, made my excuses and jumped on to the Metropolitan Line train which had just arrived, plonking myself down with a commuter on either side. She never spoke to me again.

I really acquired the whistling habit from my dad, a bricklayer by trade who would literally whistle while he worked, and from whom I definitely learned the art. Habit is, I think, the correct term, as I seem to have no ability to prevent myself from launching into whichever tune has been romping around my unconscious mind and giving vent to what in my brain is translated as a note-perfect rendering, by the magic of expelling air through my teeth, of a song which took several musicians many days of hard work to create. I can whistle it as the artist(e)(s) intended it to be heard.

At least, I believe I can. Few agree with me.

One or two of you will, I'm sure, remember this, but way back in 1967 a chap calling himself Whistling Jack Smith actually made the Top Ten with a track called 'I Was Kaiser Bill's Batman'. Yes, really. He appeared on *Top of the Pops* puckering up and whistling away, trying but failing dismally to look cool in the process. He set back the cause of we whistlers so far that we have never recovered.

The stares, stony looks and backward glances I received during the summer of 2020 whilst harmlessly walking down the road whistling shrilly and tunelessly (Metallica's 'Turn the Page' and Rainbow's 'All Night Long' were popular selections) to the detriment of folk's eardrums were tough to take. Until, that is, I realised that they weren't actually reacting adversely to my whistling talents, more being fearful that by whistling I was increasing the chances that I might be spraying them with potentially coronavirus-packed germs.

There hadn't been any government decree banning whistling nor, unexpectedly enough, was there any outbreak of anti-whistling feelings that I could detect on the likes of Twitter and Facebook, but certainly 'loud singing' had been frowned upon and ruled a red-card offence in churches, and clearly these anti-whistling frowns were related to that issue. The *Evening Standard* reported at the end of September, that: 'Bans on loud music, singing and dancing as part of new "draconian" coronavirus rules have been likened to George Orwell's dystopian novel *1984*.' I wasn't singing, loudly or otherwise, and certainly not dancing down the road, but I was undeniably whistling.

An article containing THIRTY-EIGHT things to stop doing to help avoid Covid did not contain the word 'whistling' anywhere, despite banging on about loud singing and various aspects of breathing. I really think the medics missed a trick, but as it wasn't banned, I reserved my right to do it... as, I trust, did Bryan Ferry whilst crooning 'Jealous Guy' and the Scorpions when performing 'Winds of Change'. Also, anyone having a bash at Ennio Morricone's scores for the great spaghetti westerns – in which whistling was integral to the atmosphere – after all, I can't imagine that The Man with No Name would be overly worried about contracting the virus as he went about his praiseworthy business of expunging bad guys for the general good of the world.

A few days later, I turned on my laptop, looking to see whether I had any Facebook messages: 'PROSTATE HEALER' was the message shouting at me in capital letters, alongside a picture of a dumpy brown bottle. The bottle displayed these eye-catching claims on its wrapper: 'Soothes painful urination. Wipes out urinary infections. Restores sexual function.'

This apparent wonder-brew was readily available from BensNationalHealth.co.uk in a 240mm container, and could be mine for... Before checking I had a mental guess – a fiver? No, I thought, there's probably not enough profit margin at that price. A tenner, then? Maybe, but no, probably a little higher so that 'free' post and packaging could be chucked in. So, I thought, £19.99 was the probable price.

Well, I wasn't far out. The jollop was mine for just £54.95 per bottle, albeit, I could 'subscribe to save 50%'.

I cannot deny I was tempted – tempted to contact the advertising authorities and ask whether this ad was legitimate and not just a high-quality scam, offering little for a great deal. Looking into the matter a little more deeply, I wondered how this brew was supposed to function. 'Scientifically refined ancient wisdom' was involved, I discovered. Reading on, I was told that 'the complete formula works synergistically'.

Of course it does. Sorry, I wouldn't be ordering.

24

IN WHICH OCTOBER OPTIMISM IS IN SHORT SUPPLY

NOW IT is getting personal, I thought, as I read the *Daily Telegraph* article on page two of the 2 October 2020 edition, telling me that patients would 'be forced to wait for cancer tests because laboratories cannot get hold of testing reagents [a term for the main ingredient of a chemical-based test] and kit'. This scarcity was related to problems at healthcare giant Roche.

GPs had apparently been notified that only 'the most urgent' of blood tests could be carried out, and that the 'testing bottleneck [was] affecting a host of blood tests including those for prostate cancer, diabetes, HIV and a range of heart conditions'. And there was me just having received a text from my own GP giving me details about how, once I had a date for my next telephone appointment with my oncologist, he would 'arrange a PSA test a week or so before the appointment date'... Hmm, how likely was THAT to happen now?

Just the day before, the *i* newspaper revealed that Cancer Research UK had issued a report, concluding 'earlier detection of cancer is the single biggest opportunity to save lives from the disease' and calling for significant investment in diagnostic equipment and technologies. To which I could only utter another 'hmm'. How likely was THAT to happen now?

The *Daily Mail* had also weighed in on 6 October with a two-page spread under the headline: 'As many as 36,000 lives could be lost because of delays in the diagnosis and treatment of cancer.' An associate legal director with a Bristol-based law company was quoted by the *Daily Mail* as saying that she was 'helping several prostate cancer patients who are considering taking legal action' as a result of delays to their diagnosis of, or treatment for PC during the pandemic.

The article quoted one patient who had contacted his MP when his treatment was delayed. His story was followed up on regional TV where he was seen on screen by a consultant. As a result he was referred to a fast-track service at London's Royal Marsden, where he had an MRI and biopsy, which confirmed that he needed a radical prostatectomy, which took place in August. 'If I'd had to wait four months for a biopsy, it could have been a very different story – the cancer could have spread and become incurable,' said Chris Durcan, from Birmingham, who had not been impressed when he'd been told that 'going private' could speed up his treatment: 'I got angry and wrote to people in authority, including my MP and local media to highlight the delays.' Was that not entirely understandable?

Days later, this headline certainly didn't make for comfortable reading: 'DEATH TOLLS SOAR... NOT FROM COVID' was the banner heading in the *Metro* newspaper on 20 October 2020. There were subheadings: 'DIABETES VICTIMS UP 86% IN JUST SIX MONTHS', 'PROSTATE CANCER UP 53%', 'PARKINSON'S UP 79%', 'BREAST CANCER UP 47%' and 'BOWEL CANCER UP 46%'. These were figures showing that 'the number of people dying at home from illnesses other than Covid-19 has rocketed since lockdown'.

On the same day, the *Daily Mail* brought news that 'hot needle treatment zaps prostate cancer', eye-catchingly claiming that these 'hot needles' 'fire off microwaves' which can treat PC 'in minutes'. This apparent miracle cure 'is a type of focal therapy' and involves 'high-dose energy' destroying tumours in the prostate via 'microwaves delivered through ultra-fine needles', which are inserted into the prostate through the perineum, under a general anaesthetic. And the whole procedure takes ten minutes or less.

Reportedly, 'larger' trials were due to start 'soon' at the Chinese University of Hong Kong. Undoubtedly, this treatment seemed to be garnering attention, and larger trials would certainly help determine its potential efficacy and impact.

An item in the *Daily Mail* in late October 2020, illustrated how difficult it was to increase the level of life-saving treatments available for PC patients.

Answering a question from a reader, the paper's Dr Martin Scurr wrote: 'A European screening trial that monitored men for 13 years showed that routine screening with the PSA test cut deaths by 21%. However, in order to save one life, 781 men had to be screened and 27 of them treated. In other words, the reduction in deaths was at the expense of considerable over-diagnosis and over-treatment.'

And the same paper reported on 23 October 2020, that, out of the total number of deaths in the preceding September, 861 people in the UK had died from PC, compared with 690 from Covid-19, with the highest proportion – 4,449 – dying from dementia and Alzheimer's disease, 4,014 from heart diseases and 2324 from lung cancer.

25

IN WHICH PC MAKES NOVEMBER NEWS

IN LATE autumn 2020, while others pondered whether a pandemic was suited to fireworks, I read a somewhat depressing item in the *Daily Mail* of 5 November, reporting that: 'Cancer patients' risk of dying increases by up to 10% for every month treatment is delayed.'

This was obviously referring to a prevalent feeling of the time, that the NHS was merely paying lip service to cancer and other serious conditions whilst hurling all hands to the pumps to help in the Covid conflict. This impression was only enhanced by a *Daily Telegraph* website story a week later, on the 12th:

The number of patients waiting more than a year for NHS treatment has risen 100-fold in a year, new figures show, with more than 4.3 million people now on waiting lists.

Across England, 139,545 people had waited more than 52 weeks to start treatment as of September this year – the highest number for any calendar month since September 2008. In September 2019, the figure was just 1,305.

The data from NHS England also shows 1.72 million people were waiting more than 18 weeks to start treatment in September.

A fortnight later on 27 November, a more optimistic story appeared, in which NHS England chief executive Sir Simon Stevens announced that an innovative blood test – the Galleri test, developed by healthcare company GRAIL – which may be able to detect over 50 types of cancer (including PC) was to be piloted in a 'world-leading programme', starting in mid-2021 and hoping to involve 165,000 patients, 140,000 of them aged between 50 and 79 who were 'without current cancer symptoms' but who would 'be tested annually for three years'.

More gloom a day later, as the *Times* informed us that, according to analysis of NHS data: 'The number of patients beginning treatment for cancer dropped by more than 30% in April.' However, the story added: 'By June they were above normal levels.' More optimism two days on as the *Mail on Sunday* reported that the drug Olaparib was being 'assessed for NHS use', explaining that the drug 'works by interfering with a key process that allows some tumour cells to repair themselves'. The drug was, we're told, reportedly 'highly effective' for men with hormone-resistant PC.

But, on the same day, and no longer surprising to me, the

i newspaper had the headline: 'Pandemic is delaying cancer research advances.' The story added: 'Major advances in cancer research could be delayed by almost a year-and-a-half because of the pandemic, a survey says.' That survey involved 239 researchers and was organised for the Institute of Cancer Research.

26

IN WHICH I PREPARE FOR A CRUCIAL PSA TEST

THERE WAS relief in my mind when my on and off cystitis-like effects finally subsided and I could look forward to taking the blood test which would, I very much hoped, confirm numerically the obvious professionalism of all those involved in my treatment. I awaited my appointment with the oncologist who was going to deliver her verdict on how I was.

But when the date finally came through in mid-November – for an appointment on Wednesday, 20 January 2021, at 12.10pm – the world had moved on somewhat... We were now in the coronavirus Lockdown Two phase.

The accompanying letter told me that I'd need to take a PSA test, ten or 12 days prior to the appointment, which would be (I assumed) with my oncologist, Dr A. By then, I would be some five months on from having, what I was hoping would be, my final Zoladex implant.

However, another potential stumbling block seemed to have been placed in the way of my progress towards what Dr A had hinted, when we spoke last, might ultimately be termed a 'cure'.

I had spotted a dark red substance amongst and inside my usually brown coloured stools on a few recent occasions, and in one alarming episode there seemed to be definite blood. I contacted one of the GPs at my medical centre to ask for advice. She was a little concerned, mentioned something called 'radiation proctitis', and referred me onwards.

So in November 2020, three days before my 70th birthday, I was sitting, waiting to hear from Mr Z... and wondering just how my mother must have felt 70 years ago when she knew my arrival was imminent but had no idea what sex I would be, or when I'd actually deign to appear. I'd never know, as neither she nor my dad was still alive.

I had, naturally, googled radiation proctitis, and Wikipedia told me: '**Radiation proctitis** (and the related radiation colitis) is inflammation and damage to the lower parts of the colon after exposure to x-rays or other ionizing radiation as a part of radiation therapy. Radiation proctitis most commonly occurs after pelvic radiation treatment for cancers such as cervical cancer, prostate cancer, bladder cancer and rectal cancer.'

I didn't want to know any more.

Only ten minutes after the given time of 11.45 am, Mr Z was talking me through his thoughts, which included that there was certainly a chance that I may have developed RP. He told me he'd be calling me up to the hospital – St Mark's at Northwick Park, not Mount V this time – probably to be checked out to find out for sure what was going on. So, then, another wait to find out – and I wouldn't have been surprised if I was given a date for early the next year, rather than the end of 2020.

It is difficult to explain how I was feeling about all of this – a bit pissed off, to be sure, but also not remotely surprised that it was happening. I've always believed in taking a pessimistic approach to events, on the grounds that you do at least protect yourself against nasty shocks, when you've been expecting them all along.

It had certainly seemed to be going a little too well, too smoothly, of late – everyone blithely assuming the next development would be a miracle cure. That clearly wasn't about to happen. Just because one threat had been removed, that did not guarantee that others wouldn't arrive to take its place.

This setback of sorts was, however, encouraging me to start buying records and CDs I'd always fancied but thought were a bit pricey, on the grounds that it may now be the last chance I'd have to do so... I spent a significant amount on a record I'd never previously heard, because it was a solo effort by Shirley Kent, the lead singer of a band – The Ghost – whose one LP I had acquired on release in the late '60s and had since refused to part with, despite its value soaring after it sold very few copies. I'd seen a report of a copy being sold recently for over £1100.

In early December 2020 I heard from a local MP – not in my own constituency, but the one adjoining – Gareth Thomas, who represented Harrow West, to whom I'd written upon hearing that he was conducting a campaign to ensure the continued presence of radiotherapy facilities at Mount V. These were apparently at risk of being moved some distance away, thus almost certainly leading to the dismantling of the brilliant team currently in place there.

The MP sent a lengthy response, in which he explained that he had secured a debate on the matter in the House of Commons in March as a result of which he was able to put his 'concerns' to the Minister of Health. He solved a small mystery for me by indicating that there were plans to 'invest in a new Linear Accelerator' (so THAT'S what LA stood for!) as, apparently, 'the current provision [was] nearing the end of its usefulness'.

Mr Thomas also referred to the 'great loss to my constituents', and others in the wider surrounding area, should the centre be closed, or, as he felt likely, should 'existing services' 'move into central London'. He added that 'ministers cannot confirm they will find the money to keep the Cancer Centre at Mount Vernon', and make the 'considerable investment in buildings, equipment replacement and IT connectivity' to make it fit for purpose.

Having read the Hansard transcript of the debate to which Mr Thomas referred, it appeared obvious to me that the long-term future of Mount V as a cancer centre was indeed in considerable doubt and that the most optimistic outcome may be moving the facility to an alternative local hospital in, perhaps, Watford or Harrow, rather than it being entirely outsourced at a considerable distance for many. Okay... I accepted that, as it was, many patients had to travel substantial distances and that I was extremely lucky to live so close to Mount V, but above all, my immediate concern was that by moving the centre it would take many years until its inbuilt atmosphere, expertise, history and team spirit – created literally over decades – could hope to be emulated.

Gareth Thomas was clearly not overly optimistic about the future, as in November 2020 he was promoting a petition to 'Save Mount Vernon Cancer Centre' on his website: 'Mount Vernon Cancer Centre, one of the NHS's specialist cancer hospitals is under threat of closure once again. Existing services are expected to move into central London after a devastating inquiry last year found that the hospital was so dilapidated and short of doctors and nurses that it cannot provide modern cancer care or even basic elements of treatment.'

Gareth's optimism would not have been boosted by an article appearing in his and my local paper, the *Harrow Times*, on 4 March 2021, under the headline: 'Trust backs move to Watford General Hospital'. Written by Adam Shaw, the story reported that, according to an NHS trust, 'plans to move specialist cancer services from north-west London to a hospital in Watford would be feasible'. Further information in the article suggested the West Hertfordshire Hospitals NHS Trust was 'confident' that Watford General Hospital could incorporate Mount V's current cancer services. 'There are enormous clinical benefits of having this specialist, regional service on our redeveloped site, and our clinical staff are very supportive of this proposal,' an unnamed 'spokesperson' from the Trust was quoted as saying.

The article ended by quoting Gareth Thomas as saying – accurately in my opinion – it would be a 'national scandal' should Mount V's services be lost completely.

***

6 DECEMBER 2020... 'How a jab of gel can end agony of prostate patients' declared the headline in the *Mail on Sunday*. In the item, writer Ethan Ennals explained how to combat the possibility that radiotherapy treatment directed at cancerous tissue in the prostate can also damage the rectum, sometimes irreversibly. The process would be to inject a gel into the space behind the prostate, 'which then solidifies and gently moves the position of the rectum so that harmful x-rays don't hit it during radiotherapy sessions'.

Such treatment had so far been given to very few patients, possibly because of the wide-ranging impact of the pandemic, but was now expected to become more widely available.

Having read this and other stories of advances and developments, one's natural reaction was to think 'D'oh, why wasn't that there when I was being treated?' However, logically, it was only possible to receive the treatment which was available at the time you needed treating – and there would ALWAYS be a possibly significant breakthrough just waiting to happen... tomorrow.

£45 million had been slashed from the Cancer Research UK research budget reported the *i* newspaper on 8 December 2020. 'Covid-19 has slowed down our efforts to beat cancer,' said Michelle Mitchell from the charity.

***

Anyway, an appointment had now come through for me to attend the Marlborough Suite of the Clementine Churchill Hospital at Harrow on the Hill at 1.30pm on Friday 11 December 2020, when and where I would be undergoing a flexible sigmoidoscopy. This, I was informed, was an endoscopy procedure. Feel free to google these items should you wish.

Nearer that date I was sent relevant information, and first had to attend a Covid test, which I did on a very foggy Monday morning, prior to the procedure. Seeing as the Clementine Churchill had been the scene of several injections I had undergone for trigger finger, and also the site of my two carpal tunnel operations, this was home ground for me.

I duly passed the Covid test, conducted in the Clementine Churchill carpark, so awoke a little nervously on the Friday morning, hoping that the idea of what I was about to receive might prove to be worse in the anticipation than the actuality. Part of me was reassuring – 'You'll be ok, it's just a test, they won't find anything terrible.' The other part not so – 'You've been lucky so far, law of averages says that can't and won't continue for ever.'

Just then the phone rang. It was the Clementine Churchill. 'Could you come in for 11.30 rather than 1.30, please?' That pleased me. I could hope it would now be all over before I'd even anticipated it starting.

Superstitious as ever, I dressed in what I considered the togs which would show me off in the best light – always assuming that will be a somewhat subdued light, that is.

I drove up, which ruled out the optional sedation which the pre-supplied advance information indicated as being an option if you had someone coming to collect you afterwards. There was also an alternative form of pain relief offered though – official name Entonox, better known as 'gas and air'. There was no indication about how brave you'd need to be to decline these options.

In the event, I wasn't even offered them! Perhaps I looked confident, as the only other, rather younger, patient in the Marlborough Suite with me was offered and accepted the heavy-duty alternative. He sounded very groggy on his return after being 'done' before me – he didn't even seem to want the proffered tea and biscuit. His wife arrived to escort him off the premises after a lengthy lie down (patient, not wife, that is).

Why weren't they asking me about sedation? Perhaps he was having a different procedure. I doubt it was because I looked the fearless type. Although, having said that, the lovely, middle-aged nurse who took the form I had to fill in and sign, looked closely at it, then at me, and said – honestly, I kid you not – 'You really don't look seventy.'

The next nurse I encountered said something dissimilar: 'Lie on your left side and pull your knees up, I'm going to give you an enema. Wait for at least five minutes afterwards, hold it for as long as possible, then head over to the toilet – middle door opposite. Here we go...' She sat, looking at me accusingly, after administering the dose, while I asked whether all the pelvic-floor exercises I'd done would benefit me at this stage. I swear she smirked.

Duly emptied out, I awaited the main course.

Dr Ana Wilson, a gastroenterologist, had popped in to talk me through what was to happen. Another charming, friendly lady. 'It should only take about ten minutes, I'll be looking at the left side of your colon.' This is about all I can remember of what she told me, really, but I was reassured by her.

A nice chap called Ben came in to explain that he would be pushing the bed on which I was sat into the room where I was to be flexibly sigmoidoscoped. Our affable relationship was doomed not to last that long, as he pushed me possibly 30 yards (younger readers ask your parents) into the lair of Dr Wilson.

In a refrain I'd heard before, she invited me to 'lie on your left side and draw your knees up' before inserting... Do we really need to go into gory detail? I think you can imagine what was happening at this juncture and some of those who know me well will be thinking: I wish I'd been able to do that to him...

Dr Wilson apologised for not having asked, and said, 'Would you like to watch what's happening?' For a split second I genuinely considered saying yes, but realised that I would undoubtedly faint if I did so, so politely declined.

But in a sudden reversion to the radiotherapy room at Mount V, I could hear relatively loud rock music and I recognised it as The Who, playing 'Teenage Wasteland'. I immediately relaxed and began listening closely to Daltrey, Townshend and co., to help me pretend nothing much was happening, despite the occasional little nudge or frisson in a part of me that I'd never really been aware was even there. Once The Who had finished, to be replaced by The Carpenters, the whole process was pretty much over, the cork removed, as it were, and Ben's arduous wheeling task had to be repeated in reverse. Seconds later I was back in my bay, being offered tea and rather decent biccies and told I could get dressed.

'How was it?' said the nurse.

'I think the thought of it was more traumatic than the procedure itself.'

She smiled knowingly. I was sure that's the object of the exercise.

Dr Wilson reappeared within minutes, looking pretty pleased with her work, and handed me a 'Sigmoidoscopy Report'. Under a heading of 'Procedure Comments' I read: 'Telangiectasia in the rectum consistent with radiation proctopathy – diffuse, affecting about 50% of circumference. Otherwise normal.' I wasn't quite sure about that, although the word 'normal' was encouraging.

Reading on, under a heading of 'Patient Management and Follow Up' it said: 'Discharge to GP – stop 2WW pathway. [I believe 2WW means 'two-week wait', a 'referral pathway' introduced in 2010 'to reduce waiting times for treatment of cancer, and to address the discrepancy between UK cancer survival outcomes, compared with the rest of Europe.] Patient advised on ensuring soft stool. Patient discharged (no further action required).'

At that moment I felt that I was genuinely in love with her. I was sure Sheila wouldn't mind if she read this. Not only that, but I was now in possession of several, full-colour images of my 'splenic flexure', 'proximal and distal sigmoid colon' and, prize exhibit – 'rectum'.

Dr Wilson smilingly explained I was now free to go and asked would I deliver a letter from her to my GP. 'Not before I finish my tea and oaty biscuits,' I told her.

***

The *Daily Mail* reported on 16 December 2020 that 'leaked NHS documents showed that 'the number of patients waiting for cancer tests or treatment' had risen from some 90,000 to 160,000 in just seven months. The night before, The Real Full Monty on Ice told the story of the group of celebrities, all of whom had had cancer, who were now stripping on live TV to raise awareness of cancer charities. Amongst them were rugby star Gareth Thomas, (not to be confused by the MP of the same name, campaigning on behalf of Mount V) Grand National-winning jockey Bob Champion and former 'Page Three girl' Linda Lusardi.

Two days later, the same paper reported that 'more than four million patients missed out on potentially life-saving scans during lockdown'. Jody Moffatt, head of early diagnosis for Cancer Research UK said, 'There is a cohort of patients that have not been diagnosed yet – and who knows what state they will be in when they are.'

27

IN WHICH I HEAR MY FELLOW SEDGEFIELDERS' EXPERIENCES AND MEET DR GLUM

I BELONG to a group of horse racing friends and acquaintances who decided to contribute to sponsoring a race at Sedgefield racecourse in 2010 to mark the fact that one of our number – Sean 'The Fat Controller' Magee – was completing his full set by visiting Sedgefield as the final course missing from his attendance list across England, Scotland and Wales.

I was otherwise engaged seeing family in New Zealand when this inaugural occasion took place, but it then became an annual get-together and I joined in, enjoying some splendid trips up the country, during one of which I was virtually struck dumb thanks to a nasty bug which closed down my vocal cords even as I was travelling to the track, while on another of the jaunts we all spent a few boozy hours being drunk under the table by a then octogenarian, the late Sir Peter O'Sullevan.

This group, overwhelmingly male, although 'other halves' were certainly not excluded from the gatherings, probably had an average age in the high 50s when it first assembled. A prime age, of course, for PC to emerge amongst our number.

And when I started to tell a few of my cohorts in the group about this book, I was somewhat shocked that the first three I mentioned it to all confessed, extraordinarily enough, that they were fellow victims. When I asked these kindred spirits whether they would mind sharing their experiences with me and the readers of the book, they all agreed without hesitation, repetition or deviation, as Nicholas Parsons used to instruct contestants in the radio panel game *Just a Minute*.

These are their stories.

DAVID ASHFORTH

IT SEEMS a long time ago – good, that's the main thing.

Though during the three months in the run up to November 2020 my PSA reading more than doubled to 6.7. As another three months, at that rate, would have seen it well into double figures, I was put back on hormone therapy. Now, in September 2021, I am still on it, although with my PSA down to 0.1 I will soon be taken off it again.

'A long time ago' means 2008, when I was 59, and my doctor arranged a PSA test. I have always had good GPs, with one exception. Unfortunately, he was the one that mattered. Several times previously I had seen him about peeing issues. He didn't suggest a PSA test but told me that it was just part of ageing. If I had known then what I learnt subsequently, I would have pressed him for a test. Not that peeing issues indicate prostate cancer, but at that age prudence indicates having a test.

The test returned a reading of 11.2. The doctor told me that, if it had been 7 or 8, that would have been all right but, as it was higher, it was probably advisable to see a specialist. 7 or 8 would not have been all right; it would have merited further investigation. At that time, and perhaps still, it was not only patients who needed to be better informed about prostate cancer, so did some doctors.

The next step was a biopsy. They stick an instrument up your backside to take samples of tissue from different parts of your prostate, to find out whether or not there are cancer cells and, if so, how widespread they are. It didn't take long but it was quite painful.

The results are expressed on the Gleason scale, from 2 to 10. My Gleason score was 7. I had a fairly aggressive cancer which had reached the edge of my prostate.

For me, the most difficult thing to deal with wasn't discovering that I had cancer, but the knowledge that I should have been diagnosed earlier, when there would have been a better chance of a cure. My reaction to the situation was to make myself as well informed as possible. I wanted to know the likely course of events, and the fact that nothing that has happened since has been a surprise – apart from still being alive – has made it easier to deal with. The experience of having cancer is often referred to as a battle, but for me it is not a battle but just a matter of the complex and challenging way in which prostate cancer cells behave, and the medical profession's imperfect but improving ability to treat the disease.

The specialist advised me that I needed to have my prostate removed and in October 2008 I had a radical prostatectomy. The operation took more than four hours and because the cancer had reached the edge of my prostate, surrounding tissues were also removed, which made nerve and blood vessel damage more likely. In terms of quality of life, the two main potential impacts are incontinence and impotence. Mercifully, I was largely spared the former but not the latter.

If you like penetrative sex, a radical prostatectomy can be pretty disastrous. There are some remedial options, particularly if you are prepared to stick a needle in your penis and inject a drug. In my experience it wasn't very satisfactory. On the other hand, losing erections is better than losing your life, probably. Since only prostate cells produce PSA, after the removal of your prostate, PSA readings should be close to zero. After initial readings of 0.05, by July 2010 my readings had crept up to 0.5. It's a very small number but enough for my oncologist to consider it evidence that the cancer had returned, if it had ever gone away.

From September to November 2010 I had 33 sessions of radiotherapy – 'retrieval' radiotherapy. If the cancer cells were confined to the area near the site of my absent prostate, there was still a chance of a cure. The radiotherapy itself was painless and until more than halfway through the course of treatment, I experienced virtually no side effects. At that stage the worst part of it was nothing worse than having to drink several cups of water before each session. Later on, the lining of my bowel was affected, along with my bottom, and I was glad when it ended. There is still some legacy of that.

The sessions put my own situation in perspective. When you are 61 and at the hospital you see women in their 30s, bald from chemotherapy, there are no grounds for self-pity.

After the radiotherapy my PSA reading dropped to 0.2, but by April 2011 it was 0.5 and subsequently crept up to reach 4.9 in July 2012. My oncologist, who I nicknamed Dr Glum, wrote to tell me, 'The difficulty is that we are limited in other treatment approaches apart from using hormone manipulation.' So, the following month, I started hormone therapy, which is a polite term for chemical castration.

I became fond of Dr Glum, who tended to look earnest and worried, as if he had just received some bad news. Perhaps he was about to tell me that he had a serious illness but then, instead, told me that I had.

My understanding was that, by stopping the production of testosterone, which fuels the growth of prostate cancer cells, hormone therapy would inhibit the progress of the disease but was not a cure and would only be effective for so long. Eventually, testosterone-independent cancer cells would emerge and effective treatment become more difficult.

At some point, the cancer would spread and at another point, it would kill me. In the meantime, unless something else killed me – a runaway horse, for instance – there would be unwelcome side effects. Among the rather disturbing list of items on the menu of possible side effects was putting on fat and weight, and losing muscle. I tried to find some muscles, so that I'd know if they went missing. I did put on weight and, as well as a larger stomach, notably lacking in muscles, started to grow breasts.

That was unwelcome – although resorting to the gym helped – as was the treatment's impact on genital size – making them smaller rather than larger. Perhaps to make the physical changes easier to come to terms with, my libido also shrank. It was a strange feeling. Women's beach volleyball appeared on TV and the first thing I thought was, oh, that looks like Somerset House in the background, where the Poor Law Commission used to be based.

There were hot flushes but they faded over time; there was fatigue, which was frustrating, tending at any time to replace a strong desire to do things with a strong desire to lie down. I'm not sure about mood swings, another common side effect. When you back a winner at Wolverhampton races, which then gets disqualified, your mood can swing quite a lot anyway, so it was difficult to isolate the effect of the hormone therapy. On the plus side, suggestions that the hormone therapy might only be effective for two or three years proved to be wildly mistaken. I kept a diligent record of PSA readings and treatments, partly so that I could present it to Dr Glum or other oncologists when they were busy trying to find the information in their paper files.

After receiving the first injection of Prostap (Leuprorelin), in August 2012, my PSA reading crashed down to 0.1. I had further injections every three months but when another was due in June 2013, and the reading was still 0.1, Dr Glum suggested moving to intermittent hormone therapy. He told me that this approach did not seem to shorten the period for which the hormone treatment was effective and had the advantage of alleviating some side effects. The plan was to stay off hormone therapy until my PSA reading reached 10.

So I didn't have another injection until March 2015, by which time my PSA reading was 10. It immediately went down to 0.1 and in November that year, when it was still 0.1, I was taken off hormone therapy again. I didn't go on it again until August 2018, when my PSA reading had again reached 10. Off it again in June 2019, on it again, December 2020.

As Dr Glum has been fond of reminding me, I have been lucky. My prostate cancer cells must be particularly susceptible to the withdrawal of testosterone. I'd like to think, but can't, that eventually they'll get bored and give up. After all, they can't be that clever, or they wouldn't kill their hosts.

It hasn't been an experience that I wouldn't have missed for the world, and although I'd like to report that it's changed my outlook on life and the way that I live it, the change hasn't been dramatic. I haven't been motivated to cross the Sahara on a camel or read the works of Proust rather than just carrying on following horse racing diligently, as I have been for over 50 years.

There has been more intending to travel than actual travel, but I have made a conscious effort to see friends more often and nurture friendships more. They are, I am more aware of than before, one of the most important things in life.

In the early post-operative years I was active in fund and awareness raising projects, some with Prostate Cancer UK and what is now the Graham Fulford Charitable Trust, both excellent charities. Most of the time, I don't think about my prostate cancer and when I do it's usually to think how lucky I've been and of the countless people in much worse situations. Getting prostate cancer is not unusual and there are worse cancers and worse diseases. What I hope my experience shows to those more recently diagnosed and/or treated, is that you can have your prostate removed, then have radiotherapy, not be cured, have hormone therapy, and 12 years later still be alive, active and feeling well.

I am now 71, so there's nothing to complain about. Life's enjoyable, I have a lovely partner – Patricia – to live life with, Donald Trump's no longer president and there is going racing with friends and to the pub to look forward to. Yippee!

TIM HAILSTONE

ONE AFTERNOON in October 2013, I was at the first of the Exeter Racecourse autumn meetings as duty director. But a few days earlier I had been to London to see my doctor, a very old friend, for a check-up. We had done this after the summer for many years and, every year I received a letter shortly afterwards telling me that all was okay. But this time, it was a phone call telling me that my PSA was abnormally high and that it had doubled in the course of the last year.

PSA, short for the Prostate Specific Antigen, is a protein that circulates in one's blood. It is produced by both normal and malignant cells in the prostate gland. A high level of PSA may indicate that one has prostate cancer, which, in my case, was confirmed by a biopsy.

I have never felt any pain or even the slightest bit unwell from having prostate cancer (and, indeed, it now seems quite likely that I no longer have it). It may, therefore, seem inappropriately dramatic when I say that my life changed quite profoundly that afternoon, but it is nevertheless the case.

I hadn't been properly ill in my life. I had never spent a night in hospital. I had never even had flu. Now I was a cancer patient, or, to employ a favourite media term, a 'cancer victim'. This was deeply shocking and made me feel very uncomfortable. I looked at friends who were free of cancer and felt different, even alienated, from them. For a while I, a notoriously gregarious person, even avoided social occasions.

I was 66 and had not yet stopped thinking of myself as fairly young, but now I had a disease that had the potential to kill me. I had never seriously thought about my life ending but now I realised that, cancer or not, I was already, quite probably, well into the last quarter of my days on earth.

I dealt with my sense of alienation from the cancer-free portion of humanity by issuing regular bulletins to my friends. I am not at all sure they appreciated such detailed information on my state of health but it made me feel better.

It will surprise no one that the sense of my mortality brought on by my diagnosis has remained with me. The knowledge that our days are numbered must come to all of us eventually.

There was one quite common reaction to the news that I had prostate cancer that surprised and shocked me. Quite a lot of people had the idea that prostate cancer is very slow, that you don't get it 'until' you are old and that it's rarely lethal. There is some truth in these general impressions. It is a disease of aging, prostate cancer cells grow much slower than those affected by other cancers and many men die with rather than of prostate cancer.

However, the facts are that about 9,000 men succumb to prostate cancer every year in the UK – that is a death every hour, 24 hours a day. Prostate cancer is now the biggest cancer killer of men after lung cancer.

Compared with eight years ago, when I was diagnosed, many more people now recognise what a big issue this disease is for men's health and are aware how important it is for men to monitor their prostate health by having regular blood tests.

The main agent of this change has been the charity Prostate Cancer UK (PCUK). PCUK does great work in raising funds for research, disseminating information and in supporting men who have the disease, but its most crucial contribution has been towards raising awareness.

As I got used to the idea that I had cancer, I began to feel the need to decide how to approach it philosophically. It seemed to me that I could either adopt a fatalistic approach – to do as my doctors told me, not to ask questions and let it take its course – or I could inform myself and, as far as possible, take charge of my destiny. I have one friend who took the former approach and another who took the latter. I don't believe that one is better than the other, but I knew that I needed to know as much as possible, so that I could take part in the decisions about my treatment and understand what was being done to me and why.

I read everything I could get my hands on and drove my doctor friends mad with questions. I got involved in PCUK, partly because

I wanted to support the charity but also, I confess, because it was a good way of meeting people who had relevant information to impart. Eight years later I still read pretty much everything that is published on prostate cancer and follow the major research programmes closely.

Over those eight years, a great deal of progress has been made. MRI imaging has become a standard part of the diagnostic process, so many men can avoid uncomfortable biopsies; hormonal treatments for those with an incurable disease are keeping many men healthy for many years; tailor-made, molecular treatments for individual patients are becoming a reality; and there is a real possibility that some men with advanced prostate cancer may be cured.

However, some knotty problems remain. There is still no reliable way of establishing, among men who are diagnosed with prostate cancer, those who have an aggressive form of the disease. There is a small subset of men with prostate cancer who are resistant to treatment, whose disease progresses rapidly and who die early.

I think that emergencies arising from prostate cancer are rare. The progress of the disease is slow and, although some men die, this tends to happen in a fairly predictable manner. However, I was an emergency. It happened about three months after I was parted, surgically, from my prostate gland. I was at Wimbledon on the second Monday watching the tennis on Centre Court, when I started to feel unwell. It seemed like one of those short-term 24-hour bugs, but two days later I was in hospital with septicaemia. I later learned that, for some hours after my admission, I had been dangerously ill.

When one's prostate is removed, the surgeon takes samples of some of the lymph nodes. This is to establish whether there is any cancer in them. In the great majority of patients, shortly after the nodes have been cut, they close up again spontaneously. In a very small number of patients this does not happen and the lymph nodes continue to generate lymph fluid that, by the force of gravity, finds its way to the base of the pelvis, behind the bladder. If this happens for long enough this pool of fluid can become infected and turn into something very nasty. The result is known as an infected lymphocele. When mine was drained from my body there was three quarters of a litre of it. This was the only point since I first discovered that I had prostate cancer, that my life was in danger.

DAVID HEIGHWAY

A BUPA company health check identified potential PC in June 2012: 'Your result shows a slightly raised (PSA) level which was noted in the past with no significant changes. I suggest you consult your GP about this within the next month.' The level was 6.6.

In late August of the same year, I was recommended for monitoring for three months by an Addenbrooke's Hospital urologist, which resulted in a biopsy being subsequently recommended. The biopsy was duly taken and PC found in early January 2013. The next step was an MRI scan, before a decision as to whether surgery or radiotherapy treatment would be the next stage of treatment.

At a urology clinic review at Addenbrooke's on 25 January 2013, an MRI scan revealed an 'intermediate to high' risk. I opted for radiotherapy treatment. Before this I had begun taking Casodex, a hormonal therapy.

In April 2013 gold seeds were planted in my prostate for targeting purposes. I was scheduled for 37 daily radiotherapy sessions from 3 May to 7 July 2013. I was discharged with a date for the review with my consultant, along with a PSA test appointment in three months' time.

A PSA test on 26 September 2013 showed a level of 0.10 – so the treatment was very successful. A review at Addenbrooke's on 2 October 2013 stated: 'PSA undetectable at less than 0.1. As such I have suggested that we simply touch base in six months – April 2014 – with an up-to-date blood test.'

The test in April also showed that PSA remained 'undetectable'. I was told my GP should check my PSA on a biannual basis for five years, then annually for the following five. 'Please refer him back to see us if his PSA rises above 4.0.' I was also reminded to keep my own PSA diary as I would not receive GP reminder letters.

In September 2020, after a PSA test by my GP had shown a level of 4.4, I was referred to the Addenbrooke's Urology Department in a letter dated 22 September 2020, pointing out that 'due to the Coronavirus pandemic hospitals have significant wait lists. There may be significant delays between your GP referring you and the date of your appointment.' In November 2020 my consultant recommended an 'MRI scan and nuclear scan to identify conditions of ALL organs and bone structure'. A CT thorax-abdomen-pelvis scan was undertaken on 1 December 2020 and a 'NM Bone whole body' scan precisely one week later.

The consultant called me to say the CT scan was 'clear' while the bone scan showed arthritis in some joints – 'normal aging' – and a cyst on the kidney, but no spread of PC into other organs. Next would be a PSMA scan for very specific prostate identification, locating and determining the extent of PC.

The PSMA scan was undertaken on 30 December 2020. I received a call from the consultant on 13 January 2021 to discuss the result of the scan which identified 'entrenched PC in left hand prostate (hot spot). This is concentrated and has not spread but cannot be further treated by radiotherapy, but can be controlled for many years by hormone treatment. Failure to eradicate is 4% in men treated for PC.'

The next steps were to take hormone tablets for 28 days, followed by hormone injections in the abdomen, given to eradicate PSA level to 0, which were commenced on 17 January 2021.

A DEXA bone density scan is to be undertaken within the next 12 months (probably in January 2022) at a comprehensive health check.

28

IN WHICH I IDENTIFY PROCKSTATE CANCER

OUR LIVES converged for about ten minutes back in the late '60s, but he has never written or stayed in touch... Not surprising really, I suppose – after all, Elton John is a mega superstar and I'm not.

I started reading Elton's autobiography after finding a copy in my local station's 'book exchange' freebie shelf and was surprised to read that we had something else in common – prostate cancer. I didn't recall ever reading or hearing that Elton had been a sufferer, but now here he was in the book, revealing just that.

With plans for his farewell tour 'already underway' in 2017, he found out he had cancer. During a routine check-up his doctor noticed that his PSA level 'had gone up slightly' so sent him to have a biopsy. 'It came back positive.' Told by his oncologist that he had two options – prostate removal or 'a course of radiation and chemotherapy' – he 'went straight for the surgery'. Despite potential downsides regarding bladder control and it being a major operation, Elton 'just wanted rid of it'.

His surgery took place in LA 'quickly and quietly'. Elton 'was back onstage at Caesar's Palace within ten days'. In his book he described a night in Las Vegas in 2017 when, as he was walking across the stage, he was also 'unknown to the audience, copiously urinating into an adult nappy... pissing myself in front of an audience while wearing a giant nappy... an entirely unprecedented experience onstage'.

Unfortunately, Elton suffered a rare complication from the operation, causing fluid to leak from his lymph nodes and needing to be drained on a regular basis for two and a half months, before 'a routine colonoscopy shifted the fluid permanently'. No doubt Elton will have spoken with one of his long-term pals, Rod Stewart, about their varying experiences of PC.

Every so often the media will carry a story about a celebrity who has died 'of' or 'with' PC, or who is currently 'battling' the condition or who has now 'beaten' it. Few of these go into much detail, other than the very vaguest, about how severely or otherwise the individual has been affected, and some make what might possibly be seen by fellow sufferers as slightly dubious claims. For example, in the opening paragraph of an October 2019 story about Rod Stewart in the *Metro*, which suggested under the headline 'Rod "needed radiotherapy every day in cancer clinic"': 'Rod Stewart had to have a three-month intensive course of radiotherapy because he had an aggressive form of prostate cancer, his tearful wife revealed.'

During my own treatment I was given to understand that radiotherapy is given over a maximum 39 days – requiring men to go to hospital every weekday for nearly two months. Many have just 20 days of treatment, as I found out when doing my own 39 steps, but if Rod was undergoing treatment 'every day' for three months, thus a minimum of 12 weeks, that could mean he had up to 60 treatments. Whether that was feasible or not I was not qualified to judge.

On the TV show *Loose Women* on 10 October 2019, Rod appeared via a video link with a message about PC for men – 'Guys, please get tested. Unless you go to the doctors, you don't know if you've got it. Finger up the bum, no harm done,' he declared. That's positive and did at least get the message across that testing was important.

His wife, Penny, revealed on the programme that Rod, then 74, had been diagnosed with PC two and a half years earlier. 'He wants to go on forever. He's always going for screenings,' Penny said. Rod had shown 'a few symptoms' and went for tests which revealed a problem which 'could not be ignored'. He'd been told removing the prostate gland would not cure him, so he had to undergo daily radiotherapy, 'travelling into London the same time every single day.' She said he had told nurses, when he arrived at the clinic, that this was his 'day in the office'. 'He was extremely positive,' said Penny.

During a December 2019 performance at an event for the Prostate Project and European Tour Foundation in Surrey, the 'Maggie May' singer let attendees in on his health struggle. 'Two years ago, I was diagnosed with prostate cancer,' Rod said. 'I thought this was about time I told everybody. I'm in the clear now, simply because... I caught it early.' Rod reportedly received the all-clear in July 2019.

Fellow rock star Elvis Costello was another who had been through the PC experience.

It was revealed that Elvis had been suffering from prostate cancer during early 2018 and reported that he had undergone an operation in May of that year as a result. The singer was quoted in October of that year as saying: 'It was a little upsetting to members of my family and friends about some of the hysterical versions of the reports. Tabloids in particular love to dramatise and have no sense of responsibility.'

In an interview with CBS, Elvis, born in August 1954, told his interviewer, who had asked about the 'small, very aggressive cancerous malignancy' which was removed: 'I was extremely lucky to have this little thing found... I was answering letters for three weeks – No, I am not dying.'

Then, in the November 2020 edition of rock magazine *Mojo*, Elvis opened up a little more about his experiences to interviewer Sylvie Simmons, admitting to her: 'I'm so used to being able to carry on regardless, and I just went out on the road before I had my strength back to do the job. I regret announcing it – although I had to – because people that I hadn't got round to telling personally yet got alarmed, and because other people go through so much worse... I was so fortunate to avoid serious illness. There's nothing more to say.' Elvis clearly didn't want to go into additional areas of his treatment which was, of course, his right.

It was announced on 19 September 2020 that rock drummer Lee Kerslake, who played with both Ozzy Osbourne and Uriah Heep, had died aged 73, 'following a long battle with prostate cancer'. News broke in December 2018 that Kerslake was terminally ill, with his doctors predicting he only had eight months left to live. In a February 2020 interview with BraveWords website, Kerslake said: 'I've got spinal cancer and prostate cancer – I've got it in remission at the moment. But I've also got psoriatic arthritis and osteoarthritis that's really hurting me and really painful.' He added:

When I first had it, it was 2,025 PSA [sic] – which was deadly. One of the guys said, 'Lee, you should be dead.' I must be one of those strong guys, because I just carried on, and they said, 'We're going to put you on chemo.' I had six months of chemo, and it went down to about 8.4, and they said, 'We're going to hammer this off with radiant [sic] treatment.' I went in for that and had radiant treatment every month – for six months, I think it was. And that wiped it out. So it's down to 1.2 or 1.4 at the moment.

Not every rock star diagnosed with PC survives, and another who didn't was Alvin Stardust (whose real name was Bernard Jewry, and who also had success under the earlier stage name of Shane Fenton). He had recently been diagnosed with metastatic[2] prostate cancer and died at home in October 2014, aged 72, with his wife and family around him, his manager said.

When he was recovering from his own brush with PC during 2013/14, Small Faces' drummer Kenney Jones (later also with The Faces and The Who), decided to help raise awareness of the condition with a rock concert at Hurtwood Park, his polo club in Surrey, for which he roped in a star-studded collection of rock royalty performers.

Having persuaded these participants, Kenney was approached by one star he hadn't contacted – Alvin Stardust, whose 'passion for the fundraiser surprised us', he later wrote in his biography, *Let the Good Times Roll*.

Kenney said of that time: 'a couple of months after the concert we learned that Alvin himself was battling prostate cancer. He was determined to keep his illness private. We respected those wishes.'

---

2. Some cancer cells will escape the prostate and grow quickly, spreading to nearby tissue, or 'metastasizing'.

Kenney had brachytherapy treatment for his condition, but 'the side effects were tough'; his recovery process took 'a year of discomfort and a year of healing'. 'Only after the third year have I properly felt myself again,' he wrote in 2018.

Not afraid to spread the word, Kenney wrote the following of PC in his book: 'It shouldn't be taboo. It's an illness, that's all. Get yourself tested, especially if you are over 50, even if you're not exhibiting symptoms. Don't leave it too late. One simple call could save your life.'

Frank Zappa was a controversial musician in his day. Some weren't entirely convinced that the sounds he and his band The Mothers of Invention came up with should even be described as music. Frank didn't much care what the non-believers thought and carried on creating his idiosyncratic LPs for those who 'got' it.

Sadly for me, I was never one of them, and the only one of his records I ever owned was his seventh record, *Weasels Ripped My Flesh*, released in 1970 as the follow-up to *Burnt Weeny Sandwich* – yes, really – and best described as 'jazz-fusion avant-rock'.

Frank had experienced urinary problems for some time and had himself checked out. When interviewed on American television, by which time he knew he had PC and that he was almost certain to die from it, he said, 'It's worthwhile being examined to find out whether or not you've got it. But on the other hand, over a period of years I had urinary problems and was examined, and they didn't find it. That's why it came as such a shock to me when they told me I had it, because I'd had urinary problems for a number of years.

'You can imagine how irate a person might be when you are informed that, yeah, you got it – and we can't operate on it. So, yeah, go have a test, but... get another test... get a few tests.'

Frank, finally diagnosed some two years earlier, died on 4 December 1993, just 17 days before his 53rd birthday.

Rarely, some personalities in the public eye like Kenney Jones, can feel that there is quite a lot more to say. In May 2020, Bill Turnbull was three years into a PC diagnosis, but was quoted by the *Metro* as feeling 'very, very calm' about the prospect of dying. Now aged 64, the former *BBC Breakfast* frontman, from 2001-16, had revealed in 2019 that his cancer had spread to his bones, although he was 'currently fit and well'.

In May of that year, he was interviewed by Tom Bryant of the *Daily Express*. He said: 'You can't fight cancer, you just have to deal with it.'

Turnbull was diagnosed as incurable, by which time the disease had spread to his spine, ribs, pelvis and legs. He was initially told he could expect to live for ten years. He had nine rounds of chemotherapy and hormone therapy, and radium injections to target the tumours in his bones.

Bill also utilised alternative therapies, trying cannabis derivatives to help with pain control and charting his progress in a Channel 4 documentary. He also called for changes to the law, as cannabis was, and still is, illegal in the UK. Speaking to PCUK in July 2020, before his beloved Wycombe Wanderers' successful League One play-off game – on which he was reporting – the 64-year-old said he was doing 'everything' he could 'to stay positive' and revealed he was now on his 'third different treatment'. He added that his recent results 'were very encouraging'. 'I do yoga every day, I meditate, I watch my diet and do everything I can to stay positive.' However, he added that living with cancer 'can be a burden' but that football had provided some valuable relief.

'When you have cancer, it's with you all day every day,' he said. 'Prostate cancer is a big deal because it hits so many men and the bulk of football supporters that go to matches are men,' he said. 'A lot of them are at that critical vulnerable age – 50-plus. So, it's very much in their minds.'

In September 2020, Bill, then 64, told *Mail on Sunday* writer Oliver Holt, 'One of the mantras I have is that you should try to have a moment of joy every day.' He added that he'd had 'moments of joy to last' 'for months' when he had recently been in Wembley Stadium to see Wycombe win promotion from League One to the Championship in their play-off final.

'People who have incurable diseases need a lot of psychological stuff to keep them going... it is the power of positive thinking but more than that – don't just say "I might get better" or "I can get better", but say "I will get better".

Bill reportedly gave up eating sugar and dairy products, and reportedly 'has a playlist of Tibetan chanting that brings him great comfort'. He was on new drug Enzalutamide 'that is helping him', wrote Holt, 'make significant advances against the disease that had spread to his pelvis, spine, hips and legs'.

Bill – who joined forces with fellow PC sufferer Stephen Fry to raise awareness of the condition – added that he was cross with himself for not visiting a GP for four years, when it could have been caught earlier, and now urges others to see their GP early.

The 'Fry and Turnbull effect' has been credited with leading to record levels of men getting checked for the disease and has helped raise many thousands of pounds for the charity. For instance, a Father's Day quiz for PCUK, with Fry among several other guest quizmasters, raised over £10,000.

In May 2021, then aged 65, Bill told *The Sun* that he had 'started using an £8,000 state-of-the-art oxygen chamber in a bid to prolong his life'. He added: 'I'm now on a treatment called Lutetium 177. I am also on a hormone called Zoladex. But it's just a treatment, not a cure.'

In October 2021 he underwent a blood transfusion, sharing the news on Twitter, adding: 'Can't know who gave it, but am hugely grateful to them'.

I feared the worst when news broke in late October that Bill had stepped back from his presenting role at Classic FM radio station as 'the road has been a bit bumpy recently, and I need to take some time to focus on getting better'.

Prostate cancer has to be taken very seriously in all of its guises.

In 2015, Sir Michael Parkinson received unwelcome news regarding his health, which threw his world into turmoil.

But he was told it was treatable. 'I was lucky and got an early diagnosis of prostate cancer from a blood test and got it sorted out,'

Michael explained. Speaking in the media about that moment, Michael told the *Express*: 'I closed off, didn't let my mind explore the possibilities, I just tried to take it step by step. Maybe I didn't read all the literature, but it did come as a surprise... I was lucky, my GP insisted on regular checks. It was his dedication which enabled an early intervention, so I have much to thank him for.'

Michael added: 'Millions of blokes take the view, without really understanding why they do it, that somehow it is unmanly to look after their own health. A blood test or a check-up seems unnecessary for any chap who is tough enough to face life and death as a man should. It's barmy. It's pathetic. And it's killing tens of thousands of British men every year.'

In June 2019, the *Daily Express* reported that Parky had had an operation and radiotherapy, adding that he was left surprised by some of the side effects he had suffered following the treatment: 'I didn't need chemotherapy, which was wonderful, but I had radiotherapy. It is rather remarkable to lie there doing nothing and yet to know they are destroying this thing trying to destroy you.'

Speaking about the consequences of the treatment, Sir Michael continued. 'I was not really told how uncomfortable the after-effects can be – the problems you have with the bowel or the bladder. While it's something I'd rather not have gone through, it's not life-threatening or going to make you drop dead in the street because you've got a weak bladder or whatever.'

Comedian Jimmy Tarbuck, 80, revealed in February 2020 that he had been diagnosed with PC after Tom Jones had advised him to get himself checked out. He said that he was having treatment via 'injections and tablets daily'. Advising others to follow Jones' advice, Tarbuck made a typical 'Tarby' joke: 'Boys, go for a test. It is embarrassing. The fella said to me: "We're going to give you the thumbs up." I said, "I hope not." He roared laughing.'

In February 2021 Tarby gave his support to The Royal Marsden Cancer Charity's appeal to fund a new research and treatment facility, the Oak Cancer Centre, telling the *Sunday Express*:

I had sessions of radiotherapy for five days a week over four weeks. ...They did warn I would have side effects. Some days I felt sick and didn't feel as good as others. ...I said to my team, "Well, look, if you're getting me better, I can take this... I've been taking tablets daily ever since and at the end of this month I have to go back for a check-up to see if the cancer has gone. ...I have nothing but praise for the NHS...

Another comedian, Bob Monkhouse, who died in 2003 aged 75, seemed to take a pragmatic view when he was first diagnosed. He was said to have been optimistic and determined to overcome the disease, even joking about it with his doctors, according to media reports.

His diagnosis was made after Monkhouse went for a medical check-up complaining of increasingly severe back pain. When doctors investigated, they became worried that he had problems with his prostate gland, and tests at a private hospital confirmed that he had PC.

Subsequent tests showed that the disease had spread to his bones. Monkhouse was advised that his chances of making a full recovery were very low, and urged to begin a course of aggressive drug therapy as quickly as possible. After an initial course of chemotherapy he went to rest at his holiday home in Barbados, being cared for by his wife Jackie, 66, before undergoing a second bout of treatment.

This was the second serious illness in recent years to strike the star, who won the OBE for a showbusiness career spanning half a century. He also suffered from encephalitis, an inflammation of the brain.

Bizarrely, Monkhouse appeared posthumously in a 2007 TV ad about PC, standing by his own gravestone and saying: 'What killed me now kills one man per hour. As a comedian I died many deaths, prostate cancer I don't recommend.' The ad was reportedly edited from footage Monkhouse had already shot while voiced by Simon Cartwright, a talented impressionist.

There was a link between Bob's death and that of England's World Cup-winning footballer Nobby Stiles, whose death from PC was announced at the end of October 2020.

When Nobby was diagnosed with PC, his son John spent hours researching the disease. He's also been tested and given the all-clear.

'To be honest I didn't know much about prostate cancer until dad was diagnosed. The only thing I knew was an undertaker friend of my father – he had it and he was having some treatment.

'We sort of knew he was okay and could manage it. But the first time I got wind of it was when Bob Monkhouse had it. That was a big thing. Even then it seemed a showbizzy thing. It seemed unusual to me when my dad got it but it hammered home how close it was.'

Stiles Junior became a passionate campaigner for 'Men United' – a campaign raising awareness for PC. John also became an ambassador for PCUK. He added: 'When you hear that someone in your family has got cancer it's just like a knife going into your guts. It just knocks you sideways.'

Sir Dave Brailsford, the high-profile cycling coach, who masterminded many of Britain's triumphs in the sport over the past few years, was diagnosed with the illness shortly before the Tour de France in July 2019.

The 55-year-old confirmed in a national paper interview that he had had surgery on a tumour, which doctors discovered after flagging up concerns over blood tests. *Times* writer Matt Dickinson was shown the evidence – 'a scar running five or so inches down from his navel to his nether regions' – in mid-September of the same year. Beresford described the transperineal biopsy he underwent during examinations as 'needles up your arse, basically', and having experienced the process myself, I whole – er – heartedly concur.

He eventually underwent a five-hour operation in Birmingham, from which, he admitted, he tried to recover too quickly, telling Dickinson: 'You need to heal. The only thing that can help that is time.' Brailsford said of the work carried out by the Marie Curie charity and PCUK: 'The work people do in that sector. That's touched me deeply.'

Sir Roger Moore, a self-proclaimed hypochondriac and the longest-serving James Bond actor in history – playing the secret agent for 12 years, beginning with 1973's *Live and Let Die* and ending with 1985's *A View to a Kill* – discovered he had prostate cancer in 1993. He later underwent a radical prostatectomy (removal of the prostate gland), making a full recovery, although the experience changed him forever.

In 2009, he wrote about the health scare in his memoir, *My Word Is My Bond*. 'I had plenty of time to think about my life and how close I had been to losing it,' he wrote. Moore died of cancer, aged 89 on 23 May 2017, in Switzerland.

In his 2021 autobiography, *Windswept & Interesting* (published by Two Roads), actor and comedian Billy Connolly revealed: 'I was diagnosed with Parkinson's and prostate cancer in the same week. Holy Mother of God. I got treated for the cancer and now I seem to be OK. The Parkinson's just rumbles along, doing its thing.'

A long-standing acquaintance, sportswriter and author Ian Ridley wrote an affecting piece about PC in April 2014. Here it is printed in full:

I didn't really take in what it meant when my father told me he had prostate cancer. Didn't really know what it was or understand his treatment. I just knew I was worried for him. Worst word in the English language cancer, isn't it?

But even if cancer is as likely to be random as much as hereditary, I knew too that I was probably a candidate. And so it came to pass. I did develop prostate cancer.

What I also knew, thankfully, from Dad's case was that in many cases it is treatable, especially if caught early. People recover.

The prostate gland is peculiar to men and is about the size of a walnut. It is located internally beneath the bladder, its function to help in the production of sperm.

After Dad's diagnosis, and as I entered my 50s, I began to get myself checked. It's not nice, no pretending it is, and easy to joke about. In one test, a doctor inserts a finger up the rectum to the prostate to check for signs of the roughness symptomatic of cancer. It is, however, uncomfortable rather than painful.

In my mid-50s, I began to get symptoms that I knew about from Dad: up to urinate in the night more frequently, my flow getting weaker. My PSA level – an indicator of potential for the disease taken via a blood test – had risen. A doctor reckoned I needed a biopsy.

That procedure involved a needle taking samples from the prostate, again through the rectum. Again it wasn't nice. But again, it was manageable.

It shook me when I knew I had the disease. But curiously, my shock didn't last. I don't know how or why but I was given the strength to cope. Cancer didn't actually seem the worst word in the language.

Treatments, after all, had improved and I elected for 35 days of radiotherapy – seven weeks of five days. All short bursts and painless, though it was tiring. Still, I managed to keep working.

I have to be honest and say I was more worried when it came back two years later, spreading to a few lymph nodes in my pelvis. Now there is more treatment, in the form of three-monthly hormone injections, that helps keep it under control.

More than 40,000 men a year are diagnosed with prostate cancer and one in eight of us will be diagnosed with it.

Some will die because they left it too late. One dear old friend, Bob Lucas, who was my beloved club president [when] I was chairman of Weymouth FC, ignored his symptoms, putting them down to 'old man's troubles' and I miss him dreadfully.

But it need not be that way. If this fearful, squeamish soul can go through it all and even laugh about some of it now, then so, I believe, can all men.

In his 2020 book, *The Breath of Sadness* (published by Floodlit Dreams), about the death of his wife, Vikki, from cancer, Ridley tells of the time when they were sitting next to the late, former England football manager, Sir Bobby Robson at a Football Writers' Association Dinner:

'Vikki has cancer as well,' Ridley told him.
'What type?' he asked her.
'Well, they think the primary was breast but it could have been ovarian,' she replied.
'Them, pet,' Bobby said, 'are the only two I've not had.'

29

IN WHICH I HOPE FOR A HAPPIER NEW YEAR

I AM an avid reader of, and occasional contributor to, the *Fortean Times*, which chronicles all manner of unusual and fascinating matters, even sometimes concerning the subject matter of this book. Such as the story from the Christmas 2020 edition about a 'New Jersey master hypnotist' who 'was arrested for allegedly subjecting his patients to illegal prostate exams'.

Police had launched an investigation, according to the story, after patients reported him to the police, 'describing therapy sessions during which the hypnotist had told them it was necessary to perform prostate examinations'. It was as yet unclear, said the story 'whether the patients were under hypnosis'.

The next edition of the mag reported that medical researchers using an 'advanced type of scan called PSMA PET/CT to examine prostate cancer patients' had made a 'surprise anatomical discovery, finding what appears to be a pair of salivary glands hidden inside the human head, somehow overlooked by scientists for centuries'. The research team reportedly believed that their discovery was 'another target to avoid during radiotherapy treatment for cancer patients'.

Worrying PC-related stories continued to appear as we moved towards the second month of 2021. At the end of January, this media story turned up: 'A non-invasive treatment for prostate cancer dramatically reduces side effects compared with surgery, scientists say.' This was a *Metro* story from 28 January 2021 about 'focal therapy', indicating that although it showed 'similar efficacy levels' to surgery or radiotherapy it offered 'up to tenfold reductions in urine leak and sexual problems' according to Professor Hashim Ahmed. Charity Prost8 UK was, added the item, 'raising funds for six £500,000 NHS suites' for such treatment.

A little cause for optimism there, but then: 'In the eight months from April to November [2020], 35,488 fewer patients started cancer treatments including chemotherapy and radiotherapy, down 17% on 2019,' claimed the *Daily Mail* on 1 February 2021. An NHS spokesman was quoted as saying: 'When looking at complete and up-to-date data, it's clear that the difference between 2019 and 2020 treatment is far less than suggested by this snapshot... People should continue to come forward for routine screening or get checked if they have a worrying symptom.'

I also subscribe and contribute to *The Oldie* magazine, in which I read a story by Laurence Marks from June 2020, explaining that in order to deal with the consequences of his 'enormously enlarged prostate' which involved many urgent but often fruitless toilet trips, he carried with him in his car a HeWee ('a sort of plastic receptacle in which you can have a pee on the move, or stuck in traffic'). However, it was stolen when he stopped to refuel and inadvertently left it on the car roof.

Then, having to drive home to Beaconsfield one night, he found himself 'gripped with the urge to get to a toilet pretty damn quickly'. To do so, he drove at 107mph and was inevitably stopped by police, to whom he explained: 'I have a prostate the size of a kumquat and, if you keep me here talking, I will have no alternative other than to pee all over your boots'.

They let him pee in a nearby bush and then, when he told them that his condition was bound to affect them when they were older and would 'put paid to your sex lives', they let him off, adding: 'Go on, piss off.'

Said Laurence: 'If only.'

But on 4 February 2021 in the *Telegraph*:

Health chiefs have issued a warning over missed lung and prostate cancers, urging anyone with possible symptoms to come forward for checks.

The NHS is launching a national appeal after worrying figures showed the number of people being referred for tests remains far lower than before the pandemic.

Checks for lung cancer are down by almost one third, while the number of men undergoing tests for prostate disease has fallen around 15 per cent in a year.

Matt Hancock, health secretary, was quoted: 'If you notice any unusual symptoms which last more than a few weeks, however mild you think they might be, please come forward and discuss it with your GP. The sooner you speak to your GP, the sooner a diagnosis can be made, the sooner treatment can start, and the more lives we can save.' The same Matt Hancock had highlighted his own potential risk of PC some months earlier.

30

IN WHICH I WONDER WHY ALL THE PC CHARITIES SEEM TO GO THEIR OWN WAY

THERE ARE many organisations, charities and groups working for the worthy cause of helping PC sufferers. One of the most high-profile examples is presenter Jeff Stelling on Sky Sport displaying his PCUK 'man badge'. Others are of varying size, such as Bob Champion Cancer Trust, Macmillan, Prostate Cancer Research, Prostate Cymru, Prost8 UK and The Prostate Project, to mention just a few.

Here is a little more information about some of them.

This is what PCUK have to say about their background:

The Prostate Cancer Charity was founded in 1996 by Professor Jonathan Waxman to address the 'Outrageous and arbitrary surgical treatment of men'. We were the first national organisation for prostate cancer in the UK. Our aim was to improve the care and welfare of those affected by prostate cancer, increase investment in research, and raise public and political awareness of a long-neglected disease.

We started small: five members of staff and with our helpline housed in a small room in Hammersmith hospital. It ran one day a week.

We merged with Prostate Action in 2012 and completely rebranded to form Prostate Cancer UK (prostatecanceruk.org). In the last 20 years, we've invested over £37 million into groundbreaking research, and continue to provide award-winning support for men. Over the last two decades we've funded and accelerated some of the biggest breakthroughs in prostate cancer care, from the use of multiparametric MRI to improve diagnosis, to the world's first precision medicine for prostate cancer. Both Olaparib and Ipatasertib are set to have an impact in the near future.

BOB CHAMPION CANCER TRUST

Someone tipped me off that a mutual acquaintance was involved with a charity which was actively involved in research aiming to benefit PC patients. I'd been aware that Grand National-winning jockey Bob Champion, who had himself suffered from cancer, was the driving force behind setting up the Bob Champion Cancer Trust, but I hadn't been aware of a link to PC.

I wrote to racing commentator Mike Cattermole, who I knew as a result of my work for William Hill, the bookies, to ask him about his involvement with the Trust. Mike responded:

I have been with the Bob Champion Cancer Trust for around 14/15 years now as a trustee, around half that time as chairman. We fund research projects at both the Institute of Cancer Research and the Norwich Research Park. Ours is a good little trust which tends to punch above its weight but, like everything else in this sector, we are on our uppers right now.

We are managing to keep things ticking over. The most recent achievement has been the identification of bacteria in urine which can lead to prostate cancer. Quite an exciting discovery and a paper will be published soon. It will make diagnosis easier and less invasive.

***

PROSTATE CYMRU

Started life in December 2003. Its stated aim was to create a level playing field, where men in Wales didn't need to travel to England for prostate therapies that should be available in Wales.

A national charity, Prostate Cymru is supported by fundraisers and volunteers across Wales and hopes to set up 'friendship' groups across the country.

***

THE MOVEMBER FOUNDATION

We're the only charity tackling men's health on a global scale, year-round. We're addressing some of the biggest health issues faced by men: prostate cancer, testicular cancer, and mental health and suicide prevention... We're independent of government funding, so we can challenge the status quo and invest quicker in what works. In 15 years we've funded more than 1,200 men's health projects around the world. By 2030 we'll reduce the number of men dying prematurely by 25%... We're creating positive change for men's health by raising awareness and educating men year-round, and through our take-over of the month formerly known as November.

Moustaches In Movember: 'For 30 days your moustache turns you into a walking, talking billboard for men's health,' says the publicity. Those taking part are asked to 'shave down on Movember 1st' and then let your moustache grow for the month, and 'ask friends and family to donate... Big or small, every donation makes a difference'. The promotion raises cash for 'groundbreaking health projects across mental health and suicide prevention, prostate cancer and testicular cancer'.

***

MACMILLAN CANCER SUPPORT

Macmillan is at the forefront of understanding the needs and experiences of people living with cancer. We do this by analysing public health data, evaluating services and healthcare economics, conducting surveys, funding academic research and working closely with people affected by cancer and our professionals and partners on the ground.

Macmillan's website includes a Prostate Cancer Forum: 'A place to have more general discussions and chats... [and] to discuss diagnosis and treatment.'

***

PROST8 UK

Prost8 UK is a 'new force in the fight against prostate cancer'. 'A revolutionary new force in the charity sector born from the experiences of men who have travelled different journeys through prostate cancer – some good, many not so good and, sadly too many with very early endings!'

PROSTATE CANCER RESEARCH

Prostate Cancer Research: (prostate-cancer-research.org.uk). See chapter 45 for further details.

***

TACKLE PROSTATE CANCER

Tackle Prostate Cancer: (tackleprostate.org). This is the campaign name of The National Federation of Prostate Cancer Support Groups: 'We are the only patient-led, UK wide charity representing people with PC, and those who care for them.' (National helpline: 08000355302 – info@tackleprostate.org)

***

Deciding which PC charity to support can be difficult for potential donors. It is confusing for anyone wishing to contribute towards helping to improve treatment for PC patients.

As I've illustrated, there are a number of charitable organisations looking to fund breakthrough research into the condition. All believing that their own efforts are the most vital.

How is the would-be donor to know where best to place their donation and/or support? Wouldn't we all rather see the NHS sufficiently funded to carry out such research for itself? Should we be concerned that donating money to a PC charity inevitably means that a substantial percentage of any donation might just be absorbed into general expenses, wages and operational costs, rather than directly funding relevant research?

I can't give you answers to these questions, I'm afraid. I personally know and trust people involved in raising money with which to fund new and improved treatments. They are undoubtedly genuine and committed to supporting their cause. I suspect, though, that appeals for funding will remain an integral part of the overall picture regarding research of this nature for as long as innovative and effective solutions are being sought.

31

IN WHICH I'M FULLY ALARMED

I WAS keen not to miss the appointment for my PSA test on Monday, 4 January 2021, as my prostate treatment moved into a fourth year. So anxious was I not to be late for the 7am blood-letting at my local GP's surgery that I'd set three radio alarms the night before, pessimistically still worrying that all three might fail to go off, optimistically hoping that just one would work. In the event I awoke to a cacophony of heavy metal from Planet Rock; the usual, slightly smug, patronising tone of BBC Radio 5 Live; and some terrible advert on LBC – all the alarms had functioned properly.

I hauled myself out of bed to turn the row down and avoid waking the rest of the household. I made myself a cup of tea, vaguely thinking that I should be hydrated after a night's kip, and got ready to stride out into the gloom of a damp winter's morning. Having listened to the news, I was wondering what would be going on in millions of households throughout the nation as it was the day primary schools were due to reopen... There was a huge difference of opinion between parents, teachers and their representatives, and the government as to the wisdom of allowing kids to go back, with all the obvious dangers that this carried of spreading coronavirus, at a time when the majority of the country was in a Tier Four lockdown.

I was at the door of the surgery a minute or two before seven, and after passing the doorstep tannoy grilling 'Have you been abroad? Do you have any symptoms? Are you wearing a mask? What time's your appointment?' and so on, I was grudgingly allowed into the empty building. The automatic check-in system clearly hadn't set its own alarms, as it seemed very reluctant to accept my details, though it did, eventually, do so. I sat down in the waiting room, and was joined by another mask wearer, before I was called in to be de-blooded.

A very efficient young man didn't offer me a choice, but instead had set up the chair and its arm-resting section so that I had no option but to lay my left arm on it. I'd been assuming it would be the right, for some reason.

'Make a fist, please... you'll feel a little scratch.' One could understand why the 'little prick' comment was falling out of favour.

I didn't look. Still slightly squeamish, despite a few years of being passively prodded, poked, punctured and probed.

'Hold that, please.' I duly held down the small piece of cotton wool, which was then reinforced with a couple of super-sticky plasters.

'All done. Please leave by the back door as we still have the one-way system in place...'

'Thanks for being here so that this can be done, despite everything else that's going on,' I told him. I meant it, too.

Outside it was still dark. I decided to walk down to get the papers and as I walked over the railway bridge, donning a mask to enter the shop, I was passed in the other direction by a very long-term acquaintance who just strode straight past me without a word. Wearing a mask really does disguise one's identity. How long would it take – if ever – until the majority – those realising that doing so is/was both a protection for oneself and also for the benefit of those around one – no longer felt the need to wear a mask? Or were no longer instructed to do so in various situations?

Coming back from the paper shop I began whistling, only to warn myself not to be over-confident. Yes, I thought, you've survived the injection, but you don't know what the outcome of the test will be... And then there was my 20 January telephone appointment with Dr A. Or was it? When I looked more closely at the letter giving me the date and time – 12.10pm – I noted it wasn't signed by Dr A, nor by anyone else, but at the bottom it said: 'Komal Joshi, Clinical Oncology Appointments Department'. So who knew who would be doing the phoning...? Not me!

Later in the day, our glorious leader, Mr Johnson, appeared on TV at 8pm to announce in true *Groundhog Day* fashion that we were to return to a third lockdown situation, in an effort to restrain the surge in Covid cases, coinciding with the roll-out of the second vaccine. Oh, let joy be unconfined – as it had been just minutes earlier when Sheila and I had finished our daily evening watch of the excellent Netflix chess-related series *The Queen's Gambit*.

The too-early whistling came back to haunt me when I received the anticipated letter from my GP's surgery, in which I expected to be informed of my current PSA level. It began: 'Your recent blood test showed a slightly raised potassium level. This often occurs when the weather is cold. Please arrange a repeat blood test at the surgery.'

What?! Potassium? What's that all about – and where was the PSA update? If this wasn't bad enough, I also learned the following:

'Your cholesterol is raised. You may benefit from cholesterol lowering medication...' Bloody hell, what was going on?

It wasn't until the next day that I was told that my PSA level was 'normal' at 0.01. Finally, some encouraging news. Although whether that was still the effect of the three-monthly implants not yet having reduced, I wouldn't know – but Dr A would.

I'd been allocated an imminent telephone appointment, too, when I hoped to find out when I'd be going to die of excess potassium and cholesterol and whether I would have to go ahead with another blood(y) test.

I was mentally writing off the continued use of butter, sausages, cream and biscuits... but thought I might as well have some for the final time, so that I'd be able to remember what they tasted like.

The GP duly rang and explained to me that my 'potassium' result would indeed need re-checking. 'The blood goes off to a lab to be tested and we've found that during cold weather the potassium results can come back high,' she said. 'So can you book another appointment?'

No, I didn't bother to point out that it was quite likely that in the current depths of a chilly, frosty January, it was going to be just as cold next Monday as it was when I had the original test, so wouldn't the result still be...? And what about the cholesterol?

'Well, given your age and the "7" you scored in the blood test I'd recommend statins. How's your blood pressure?'

'Fine as far as I know, it has been whenever I've had it taken before, anyway.'

'Ask them to do a BP check when you have the blood test,' she said. 'You could have an 18 per cent chance of a heart attack.' That's about a 5/1 chance in bookmaking terminology.

'What, presumably not during the blood pressure check, though?'

'No.'

Right, on to the phone to book the tests. A pre-recorded message told me I was 'Number One' in the queue to be answered. Great. Then it cut me off.

I rang back. 'You're number one in the queue,' I heard again. Right, I thought, I'll double my chances of getting through and ring on my mobile...

'You're number one in the queue.' How could they have two number ones?

One of them eventually answered, but I still seemed to be 'number one' on the other line. Oh well, I was booked in for 9.34am on Monday. Very precise. My excellent PSA level barely got a mention. I'd take that up with Dr A. A text from my GP told me on 6 January: 'I have reviewed your PSA result and I am pleased to inform you that it is normal.' Yes. 0.01, I know. I'm happy with that as well.

The day before my latest blood test, the *Sunday Telegraph* was revealing: 'NHS hospitals are treating less than half of the cancer patients they normally would, it has emerged amid increasing fears it is struggling to cope with surging coronavirus cases.'

I did get in for my appointment at not much past 9.34 – having swallowed down *two* cholesterol-reducing drinks beforehand. The gentleman doing my blood test was the same one who had done the last one a few days previously. He looked at me a little quizzically (albeit that might have just been down to the mask), as though he vaguely recognised me. He wasn't phased when I asked to be jabbed in the right arm as the left was still a little bruised from last time.

After that he duly took my blood pressure, twice commenting: 'That's good. Good.' I decided not to ask him to make sure my sample was wrapped up warm en route to whoever would be analysing it.

It was, though, a little less cold than it had been the previous week, so perhaps that would turn out to be a good sign...

On the morning of Tuesday, 12 January, sat waiting for a call from a proctologist, I read this from the *Telegraph*: 'Advanced prostate cancer sufferers are 16 per cent less likely to die if they are heavy coffee drinkers, a study in the British Medical Journal has found. Every cup of coffee drank could reduce prostate cancer risk by as much as one per cent, according to researchers at the China Medical University.'

Leaving aside the fact that I rarely drink coffee, and my admittedly poor grasp of advanced mathematics, but was this second paragraph telling me that if I drank one hundred cups of coffee, I would have reduced my chance of getting PC by 100%? That was clearly nonsense.

Much more feasible was the report in the *Metro*, suggesting that researchers have found that 'regular consumption (of coffee) reduces the chance of getting the disease by about 10%' and also cuts the risk of tumours spreading beyond the prostate by 12%.' It added: 'coffee drinkers with advanced prostate cancer were found to be 16% less likely to die than other seriously ill patients.'

There was some other support for the research quoted:

Professor Nick James, a prostate and bladder cancer research professor at the Institute of Cancer Research, said chemical processing may also be responsible for the correlation that the study discovered.

'This is something that has more credibility than most food association stories,' he said. 'People will be more accurate in their levels of recall about the amount of coffee that they drink – it is a habit that people get into.'

I was not sure that I would abandon my tea-drinking habit, though.

As I may have mentioned before the trouble with this type of 'research', is that by its very nature it makes anyone reading it in a positive way feel disappointed that it has appeared AFTER they've already acquired the condition from which they are now informed it could have protected them.

And what it also doesn't usually reveal is just how far into the future these positive findings can be put into regular use for those who could benefit from it. So, in a way, I rather thought it would be better if the population as a whole were not informed of such things until they were ready for use.

All of which just emphasised again what a debt we all owe to the geniuses (genii?), oh, clever people, who broke the sound barrier to produce Covid vaccinations. Respect to them all.

On 15 January, I came across a PC reference online:

Our biological or circadian clock synchronizes all our bodily processes to the natural rhythms of light and dark. It's no wonder then that disrupting the clock can wreak havoc on our body. In fact, studies have shown that when circadian rhythms are disturbed through sleep deprivation, jet lag, or shift work, there is an increased incidence of some cancers including prostate cancer, which is the second leading cause of cancer death for men in the US. With an urgent need to develop novel therapeutic targets for prostate cancer, researchers at the Sidney Kimmel Cancer [Center] – Jefferson Health (SKCC) explored the circadian clock and found an unexpected role for the clock gene CRY-1 in cancer progression. The study was published in *Nature Communications*.

No, I didn't really understand what that meant, either.

It was now three quarters of an hour past the time, on 20 January, that my proctology call was scheduled to have happened, but it hadn't. I had, though, received a message from a friend of many years' standing, who I knew also had PC:

I have a secondary, Graham. It means my cancer has spread and is in my pelvic lymph nodes and there is no cure element now, only life extension. I am on hormone drugs and steroids, plus six-monthly injections [*sic*] of another hormone – not quite high enough risk for the first wave of vaccines. I have been having bloods every month for PSA and other levels due to the steroids, switched to three months from December.

He wasn't asking for sympathy in telling me this, although I did of course feel extremely sympathetic upon reading it. He also told me that he wondered why people like himself, and many others, who were receiving regular injections for PC and other conditions, could not also be given Covid jabs at the same time. An idea with some merit, I'd have thought.

The call referencing my sigmoidoscopy procedure was eventually almost an hour later than advertised but I genuinely did not mind. I understood how busy they must have been, and during the last few years that I've been undergoing treatments of many kinds, as you have been reading, the dates and times I have been given have, so far, been generally met efficiently. I have come to think that an appointment kept on the promised day is acceptable; within a couple of hours of scheduled time is worthy of complimentary comment; and within a few minutes deserves high praise!

'There's nothing sinister that we can identify,' I was told, and advised to keep a watching brief and if I noticed anything untoward, to draw it to their attention. I later received a copy of a letter sent to my GP from someone signing off as an, or the, 'RSO' about this procedure: 'I am pleased to inform you that the flexible sigmoidoscopy... showed no sinister pathology. He does have changes consistent with radiation proctopathy and was given some advice to maintain soft stools.'

I have taken that advice to, well, heart, though not an accurate bodily reference, but it isn't as easy as you might think – not that, I'm sure, you have ever given such a matter the slightest consideration. I was also informed that if it did 'become problematic in the future there [were] treatment options such as Sucralfate enemas'. I didn't like the sound of that, so was hoping for an unproblematic future...

I received a slightly confusing text from my GP's surgery, which became clearer when I read in the *Daily Mail* that: 'Family doctors have been told to stop routine appointments... most surgeries should pause non-urgent appointments such as health checks, routine blood tests and medication reviews.' Hmm. I'd had my blood test but did this mean the results wouldn't be immediately forthcoming, I wondered...

Saturday's *Telegraph* didn't increase my optimism: 'GPs have been told to stop much of their routine care because of the pressures of the coronavirus pandemic.' This, I suspected, might well explain why I had still to receive any information about the results from Monday's retaken blood test as of yet, when the results from the initial test had appeared within about 48 hours.

Now I was wondering whether my scheduled appointment with Dr A in four days' time could be under threat. However, she wasn't a GP, so I rather hoped not.

I'd given up expecting a text from my GP about the retaken blood test, but decided on 19 January to check whether the results would appear on my personal section of the surgery's website and sure enough they did – potassium 'normal'!

This was nearly as exciting as reading in the *i* newspaper that 'celebrities from the world of entertainment, sport and business [were] lining up to jump in a piddle' – oh, sorry, that's *puddle* – 'in a bid to raise £1m to fund research into cancer'.

Was there no end to people's willingness to undergo terrible privations to help Cancer Research UK to raise dosh? Evidently not and – removing my cynical hat – I could only welcome their puddly pluck.

Given my 46 years of working for a bookmaking company, it was somehow appropriate that on Wednesday, 20 January 2021, Dr A should ring me at 20 to one, to tell me: 'I have your most recent PSA test result. As far as I'm concerned, you're absolutely fine. I'll check in with you every six months, and send you a form to take a PSA test...'

As if that wasn't enough good news, she confirmed it in writing to my GP, who sent me a copy of her letter: 'His recent PSA was entirely satisfactory measuring less than 0.01. He had a recent flexible sigmoidoscopy which showed some changes related to his previous radiotherapy and this has now settled. Overall I am delighted with his progress and I will look forward to speaking with him again in six months' time.'

And me, her...

32

IN WHICH I'M MARCHING FOR PC

BY NOW I already knew the precise date and time when I'd next have cause to speak to my oncologist, having very efficiently been sent a very precise notification via post dated 26 January 2021 that: 'We will contact you on Wednesday, 21 July 2021 at 11.10.' If all went well, I intended to be on holiday in Jersey by then, but as I'd be accompanied by my phone it should not prove to be a problem.

The date the letter was sent to me was also the day on which I received my first Covid vaccination, which was administered on a very chilly morning, at Barnet FC's ground, The Hive, on 26 January 2021. For the benefit of unjabbed readers, this is what happened. I had the AstraZeneca version and the whole experience was very efficiently run. My son, Paul, drove me there. We arrived a little early for the appointment but were told it was quiet, so I should go through now, which I did.

Confirming my details at the door to what I assume was normally the club's bar, I then walked through and was directed to a desk with a waiting doctor – there were six or eight such desks. The doctor asked whether I had any allergies or other medical problems, explained about the vaccination I was about to receive, asked if I had any questions, asked which arm I'd like to receive the jab and promptly delivered the dose.

I was then asked to sit down for ten minutes just to ensure there was no adverse reaction, which there wasn't, and then I walked around the pitch area and back to the car park. All done and dusted in about 15-20 minutes.

Overnight I had a low-level headache and felt generally a little achy, but didn't have to resort to paracetamol or any other tablets. The next day I was okay but felt I was operating at about 90 per cent capability. The day after, I was completely back to normal. No anti-vaxxer, me. And, yes, I would support compulsory injections for everyone given the current situation, other than those with genuine medical reasons not to be vaccinated. I was given a small card confirming the date and the batch number of the AstraZeneca jab I had received, with room for details of the eventual follow-up stabbing to be entered.

I had mixed feelings when it came to my attention that PCUK was organising a March the Month fundraising exercise in that month of 2021. The idea was to sign up to walk 11,000 steps per day for the duration of March, and to invite people to sponsor you for so doing in order to raise funds for PCUK: 'March the Month is a virtual walking challenge everyone can get involved with. Walk 11,000 steps a day throughout March for the more than 11,000 dads, partners, grandads, sons, brothers, uncles and mates who die from prostate cancer every year. Sign up and raise money to fund lifesaving research.'

Of course, a charity of this nature needs to encourage people to fundraise to support their very worthy activities. However, I did not, and would not, feel comfortable using emotional blackmail on friends and acquaintances to hand over dosh to any cause, no matter how worthy, just because they know me and vice versa.

I also think that such ventures can often slip into virtue-signalling territory from some of those participating.

So why volunteer to take part, then? Partly because I would happily donate a few quid of my own, which I am confident will be going towards an organisation which undoubtedly does positive work on behalf of PC sufferers. Even if, again, I am a little uneasy about what percentage of the money raised by charity promotions pays hefty salaries for some of those working for charities – prime example, someone like David Miliband.

Running these thoughts about charity walking past some acquaintances produced mixed reactions. Near-neighbour Gordon, a trusted sounding board, offered: 'I have some strong opinions about fundraising, centred around why people will only give if someone half kills themselves climbing Ben Nevis backwards and wearing a suit of armour.'

My sister Lesley still wanted to donate, saying, '[I] understand your feelings but would happily donate because of you having had it.' She added it was also because a close relative of ours had had testicular cancer. She did make the caveat: '[It's] always difficult to know how much of a donation actually reaches where it's really needed.'

Brother Barry: 'Happy NOT to donate to either PC UK or Luton Town season ticket [the alternative I'd generously offered him]. I do agree there are issues about "where the money goes" within charities but will add something to our annual donation to Willow [his own family's pet charity] in recognition of your efforts.' That's great – yes, if you want to donate BECAUSE of me, do it for some cause close to YOUR heart. Absolutely.

By the way, I checked Mr David Miliband's Wikipedia page, which declared that the former Labour MP was 'a British public policy analyst who is the president and chief executive of the International Rescue Committee [IRC]. He was the Secretary of State for Foreign and Commonwealth Affairs from 2007 to 2010 and MP for South Shields from 2001-13.'

His salary in October 2019, I read on the *Daily Mail* website, was a pay package of $911,796 (£741,883) according to the US-based organisation's latest tax return, given to him as chief executive of International Rescue Committee. In late October 2021, the *Mail on Sunday* reported his annual salary as £786,000.

On their website I read that the IRC has a 'Mission to help people whose lives and livelihoods are shattered by conflict and disaster to survive, recover and gain control of their future.' Laudable, I'm sure, and if Mr Miliband had volunteered selflessly to help them on an unpaid basis, I might have been prepared to chuck them a few quid. But...

Anyway, I seem to have strayed from the subject in hand, or on foot, of Marching the Month. Having done a lockdown walk a couple of weeks earlier with pal Les Hawker, who had told me that we had walked 10,000+ steps when we returned to our starting point, I figured that, actually, walking 11,000 a day was very achievable. Making sure one did so every day of the month might have practical consequences, but given that we were unlikely to be out of lockdown before then, it seemed worth having a go at.

Let's see how I get on, I thought. I reckoned I was slight odds-on to achieve the stated aim. Don't worry, I'll come clean here about whether I managed it!

I got off to a decent start by managing to install a 'steps app' on my phone... No, okay, of course I didn't... my son Paul did it for me.

I tried it out on Valentine's Day, Sunday, 14 February 2021, and by the end of the day I'd done over 9,000 steps just by doing effectively what I had been doing every day since the first lockdown began, so I was already figuring this was not going to be too taxing a target to complete on a daily basis.

Having completed a couple of weeks since having my first Covid jab, Sheila had decided it was now once again my role in life to undertake the supermarket shopping. So I was packed off to Waitrose bright and early one February morning, arriving at about ten past eight.

Wandering blearily into the branch I was offered a splurge of hand sanitiser by a helpful member of staff who, whilst pumping the gunge on to my hands, peered closely at me and asked: 'Aren't you the chicken man?'

'Er, yes, I'm afraid so...'

'I heard all about you – you shouldn't have brought it back.'

'I'd do the same again in the unlikely event that such a thing should ever reoccur. Besides, had I not, having probably been caught on one of your security cameras, you'd probably have put Wanted posters up and arrested me this morning!'

The week before I'd been in this same Waitrose buying a few items including a free-range, corn-fed chicken. On returning home I'd unloaded my booty in the kitchen. 'Where's the chicken?' demanded Sheila. Checked shopping bag. Empty. No chicken. Must have left it at the checkout.

Drove back to supermarket. Asked the lady at the checkout, 'Did I leave my chicken here?' 'I don't think so,' she replied. I asked one of the supervising ladies if anyone had handed in a chicken. She said no, but, recognising me as a regular, invited me to take another from the shelf. So I thanked her, and did so. Chucked it in the boot. Took it home. Opened the boot, to see two chickens sitting there.

I took one back to the shop. Handed it to the bemused supervisor, whilst apologising profusely. The small audience of amused staff and shoppers debated whether they could now put the chicken I had just returned back on display. They decided not. 'You probably should have just kept it and said nothing.'

Now feeling guilty for being honest, if stupid, or, perhaps, vice versa, I made my apologies and excuses and retreated, humiliated and doomed to be known in future as 'The Chicken Man'...

***

Once again the persistent reminders that the ongoing focus on coronavirus by the authorities was absolutely damaging cancer treatment was emphasised by the *Daily Mail*, in their Comment column of 19 February 2021: 'Britain faces a "cancer disaster" leading to 35,000 needless deaths – many heartbreakingly young – due to delayed treatments and operations.' A two-page spread revealed that 'Experts say funding is urgently needed for equipment such as advanced radiotherapy machines, which provide treatment more quickly, to help doctors clear the enormous backlog'.

This was backed up by oncologist Professor Pat Price, founder of the Catch Up With Cancer campaign: 'Newer radiotherapy machines can do one round of treatment in 15 minutes, whereas older models take 45 minutes. That means you could treat three times as many people.' He didn't elucidate on whether, or how, this would be a huge improvement for PC treatment in particular. After all, my own treatment sessions had only taken about 15 minutes each...

On the same theme, Professor Angus Dalgleish, an oncology specialist at a London teaching hospital, highlighted a possibly under-mentioned aspect of the situation: 'the incidence of cancer patients themselves cancelling their scheduled hospital operations because they fear catching Covid.' This, he warned, leads to people 'sacrificing their own health and fuelling the cancer nightmare'.

Interesting stuff. Obviously I couldn't know how I'd have reacted had my own treatment coincided with the pandemic. There would have been clear pros and cons to consider.

Obviously, PC does tend to affect older men, who have also been some of those at greatest risk from Covid. The hospital where I was treated wasn't a general hospital and it didn't have an A & E unit, so probably the majority of patients would have been aware of the risks to themselves and been taking steps to minimise both them, and their risk to others.

The big problem would clearly have been mingling with the others in the waiting rooms which, I had been told, had been eliminated during the pandemic. That would seriously have diminished the experience which I had had – although, had non-mingling been in place from the start I'd never have known that, anyway. I probably would never have met Ron, again, not then knowing that it would be a good thing to meet him! I also suspected I'd have been more worried about PC than Covid and would have opted to attend as advised by my GP and oncologist. But I doubt I'd have been inspired to write this book.

***

Coincidentally, even as I was typing these words, our excellent and conscientious postman, Luigi, strode down the driveway to deliver today's mail mayhem – which included, I soon noticed, a missive from The Institute of Cancer Research: 'Cancer research must not stop for the coronavirus. Please help us bring personalised treatments to children with cancer.'

33

IN WHICH I STEP UP

ON 19 February 2021, I walked 14,016 steps, my magic, step-counting device indicated, so I now knew, pretty much, how much walking I would need to do each day during March to achieve the required amount to complete March the Month. It wasn't going to cause me much angst.

***

On Monday, 22 February there appeared in the *Daily Telegraph* this article:

Cancer death rates will fall this year despite warnings that the Covid pandemic has brought treatments to a 'screeching halt', a study has predicted. Researchers forecast that there will be some 176,000 deaths from 10 major cancers in the UK by the end of the year, with rates falling overall. The scientists said their findings correspond to death rates of 114 per 100,000 men, which is down 7.5% since 2015, and 89 per 100,000 women – down 4.5% from then.

The paper, published in the *Annals of Oncology* journal, focused on cancer of the stomach, intestines, pancreas, lung, breast, uterus (including cervix), ovary, prostate and bladder, and leukaemia for men and women. Researchers predicted that some 69,000 cancer deaths will be avoided in the UK this year.

No, I didn't know what to make of that somewhat counterintuitive article. But then, I supposed, figures can be made to mean whatever one wants them to suggest. And it was only a prediction...

A remarkable story turned up on the BBC News website, written by one Charlie Jones, who explained that: 'Dogs can detect the most aggressive forms of prostate cancer and could help develop a "robotic nose" to find the disease in the future, a study says.' 'Under an international research programme,' revealed Mr Jones, 'a Labrador, Florin, and a vizsla [a Hungarian breed], Midas, sniffed out the cancer's odour in urine samples from patients. They were trained to find the most lethal tumours by Medical Detection Dogs, a Milton Keynes charity. Clare Guest, the group's founder, said... "The dogs have been able to identify these very aggressive cancers. This could lead to lifesaving work in the future that would enable us to understand the difference between other diseases of the prostate and those that will go on to kill men," she said.' Clare went on to predict that the dogs could save '"millions of lives around the world" if they were used to support the current detection method for prostate cancer.'

Mr Jones continued:

Results from the study, backed by the Prostate Cancer Foundation and published in the journal *Plos One*, showed the dogs correctly identified positive samples 71% of the time when detecting the most lethal prostate cancers... The charity said work was also under way on a 'robotic nose' – an electronic device that replicates the sniffing ability of dogs, which would eventually take the form of a smartphone app... Dogs from the charity are also being trained to sniff out coronavirus and could be used at airports to screen people arriving from abroad, with results from the trial expected soon.

Checking for other reports about these potentially doggedly impressive results showed that the idea had been around for a number of years with a May 2014 article claiming that according to Italian researchers: 'Dogs can sniff out prostate cancer with uncanny accuracy.'

I was saddened to read, in the *Racing Post* on 24 February, of the death of Irish racehorse trainer Tom Foley at the age of 74.

The paper called him 'one of the gentlemen of Irish racing' adding: 'He had been battling prostate cancer for the last few years.'

You will already be aware of my thoughts on the term 'battling' in this context. However, I remembered fondly the very classy jumper, Danoli, which Foley had trained during the 1990s. He raised the roof at the 1994 Cheltenham Festival when he was regarded as the Irish 'banker bet', and duly obliged in the Sun Alliance Novices' Hurdle under Charlie Swan. Danoli won 17 races, including the 1997 Hennessy Gold Cup at Leopardstown.

***

On 1 March I began my quest to support the March Into March campaign with a daily score of 11,643 steps. This only meant a couple of changes to my two daily walks, and I was ahead of schedule. It stayed that way on day two, as I managed to clock up well in excess of 12,000 steps with the assistance of Sheila who was happy to walk with me. I now began to realise that either the app I was using was set too generously in favour of my steps, or I had seriously overestimated the potential difficulty of achieving the daily score.

Even as I strode into day three of this, er, stepathon, I was concerned by a *Times*' article headed 'Think again on prostate drug, plead charities'.

The story said that not only PC charities but also 'experts' are asking the National Institute for Health and Care Excellence (aka

Nice, possibly a misnomer) to 'reconsider its rejection of a drug that could extend the lives of 2,500 men each year.' The drug in question, abiraterone, which I have drawn to your attention previously, was, said the story, 'available to patients in Scotland'.

The drug cost £35,000 a year 'privately' and was approved for those who have had chemotherapy or have stopped responding to hormone drugs. According to PC UK it 'had been shown to extend life by an average of 15 months if given to men earlier, a crucial factor for those who cannot have chemotherapy'. Such treatment had, added the story, been authorised temporarily during the pandemic.

A NICE spokesman was quoted as saying: 'Abiraterone does not represent a cost-effective use of NHS resources for people at this stage of the treatment pathway.'

The article was clearly influenced by a prominent missive on the 'Letters to the Editor' page, bearing the signature of many medical professors and representatives of PC charities such as PC UK's chief executive, Angela Culhane, and Ken Mastris, chairman of Tackle Prostate Cancer, and also by professor of oncology, Jonathan Waxman.

One's immediate reaction was to bemoan the use of the phrase 'cost-effective use' and to think, this didn't sound like a vast amount of money. But then we have to accept that there are many other equally 'worthy' causes reliant on NHS funding – which is not an infinite amount. Someone, somewhere, was also no doubt responsible for quantifying effectiveness by survival time gained, and maybe they pondered, then concluded that 15 months was not a great deal, but thought, well, if it were two years plus, we might well be able to justify the cost.

Journalist and author Ian Ridley lost his wife to cancer and is a PC sufferer himself. He made his view public on his Twitter feed: 'I'm fortunate to be on the amazing drug Abiraterone, which extends life for those with advanced prostate cancer. It is being denied to too many men.' He also requested that anyone reading this or following him on Twitter should support a PC UK campaign to make the drug more readily available. As ever with the PC UK website, I found it a little difficult to find the right page for adding one's name to the campaign, but I managed to find it eventually as, apparently, had 10,818 other people – which did rather suggest that it was me at fault, rather than the PC UK website! However, I do feel I have to say what a maze the PC UK website always seems to me. I accept that this could just be me and my inability to find my way around it. But I'm not entirely stupid, and I was pleased to have become involved in the March Into March project, yet day after day it took me a considerable amount of time to find a way to access my own page in order to log my up-to-date total of steps.

Still treading the streets to clock up my 11 grand's worth of steps per day, I checked in to register that day's score when I spotted a video by Lauren Clark, the widow of cricketer Bob Willis, about Bob, his career and his death due to PC – which is dealt with in more depth elsewhere – and her eagerness to raise awareness of the condition and its dangers.

In the video Lauren tells viewers: 'I can't get prostate cancer, but like too many wives, partners and families, I couldn't have been more affected by it.' She spells out the need for speedy action when PC is diagnosed:

One in eight men get prostate cancer; one in four black men get prostate cancer. It's a very, very big problem. You're more likely to get prostate cancer if you have a history of it in your family so you must take that very seriously.

I urge men, and their wives and partners, to join the fight to stop prostate cancer killing men unnecessarily, and far too young. It doesn't have to kill you, but if you leave it too late it can be devastating.' And Lauren adds that: 'I want Bob to have a legacy, to try and help save men's lives.

It is a moving and emotional piece of work and it only enhanced the admiration I had felt for Lauren since first speaking to her. It also gave me the idea of contacting her to ask whether she'd let me use an image of the painting of Bob, which she was inspired to create following his death, in the book. She's quick to respond: 'Of course you can reproduce the image.'

She made the image specifically of Bob's bowling action, which she has captured perfectly, whilst leaving his face a blank, and, interestingly, in the video she also shows the viewer another painting at Lord's, which depicts Bob amongst some of his cricketing contemporaries. However Lauren comments that: 'I'm not sure it really *is* Bob, it doesn't look all that like him. I think he thought it was a bit embarrassing, actually.'

Perhaps, though, this reflects the way in which we all have multiple images, and all see each other differently, and just how difficult it is to call to mind an exact image of what a deceased loved one really looked like. After all, we all look entirely different depending on the circumstances in which we find ourselves. Lauren's decision to focus on the bowling action ensures that every cricket fan of a certain age will instantly recognise and associate it with Bob, thus being able to bring to mind their own favourite image of the man's face when viewing it.

34

IN WHICH THERE IS HOPE THAT THE PANDEMIC COULD BENEFIT CANCER TREATMENT

THIS FROM the *Daily Telegraph*, 8 March 2021:

Despite promises at the start of the crisis that patients would be unaffected, more than three million people in the UK have missed cancer screenings as a result of Covid.

A recent study suggested that NHS hospitals were wrong to tell cancer patients to postpone treatment during the first wave, as even those who were immuno-compromised had a better chance of survival by continuing with their treatment than postponing it, even if they caught Covid.

Four days later and the same paper was reporting:

The number of men given an urgent referral for suspected prostate cancer has fallen by more than a quarter since April 2020, new NHS figures show.

Health officials urged any men experiencing possible symptoms of the disease to come forward for help, with warnings that lives are at risk.

NHS data shows that last year, the number of men starting treatment for the disease was a third down on the previous year, with 8,600 fewer men treated.

And the number of patients referred for suspected urological cancers fell by 28 per cent between April 2020 and January of this year, compared with the previous year. It means around 52,000 fewer patients were referred.

Experts said thousands of men could be missing out on potentially life-saving treatments, suggesting the decline was because men were less likely to have consultations with their GP after the country entered lockdown.

***

My daily routine – which I had realised had been so important to me during the PC years – was to be disrupted on Monday, 15 March 2021, when I was required to deliver Mrs Sharpe to the Edgware Community Hospital Breast Screening Unit. The Community Hospital appeared to be all that was left of Edgware General, which was on pretty much the same site and is actually where I was born, although on arrival I was given to understand that no plaque marks this fact.

Returning to the importance of routine – today we were unable to take our usual 1.45pm seats in front of the TV to watch an episode of *Doctors*, which for four days of the week (it isn't on on Fridays) marks the dividing point between morning and afternoon activities. The latter had recently been able to happen following *Doctors* but before *The Bidding Room*, which comes on at 4.30, but now that had been taken off air and replaced by *The Repair Shop*, of which I was not that big a fan – too many predictable gasps of incredulity, washed down with pre-prepared tears when the previously beat-up old object was unveiled in its new pristine condition, which effectively made it something completely different from what it should be. After all, if returning something to its original condition was the object of the exercise, why not also give plastic surgery to the owners of the items, restoring THEM to the appearance they had had when they obtained these, usually underwhelming, things?

I found some PC news via an American source, advising that: 'A urine test based on University of Michigan Rogel Cancer Center research could have avoided one third of unnecessary prostate cancer biopsies while failing to detect only a small number of cancers, according to a validation study that included more than 1,500 patients. The findings appear in the March issue of the *Journal of Urology*.'

Meanwhile, the *Daily Mail* informed me that 'Macmillan Cancer Support estimates that 37,000 more patients should have started treatment for cancer between March 2020 and the end of January 2021'. A comparison of numbers for January 2021 with the same month in 2020, added the *Mail*, 'showed an 11% drop in the number of patients being seen by a specialist for suspected cancer following an urgent referral'.

I could empathise with anyone in that situation, as I knew just how I would have felt in their shoes.

Shortly after reading this item, I received an email from my almost-local MP, Gareth Thomas, with whom I had been communicating for some while about whether the Mount Vernon Hospital was going to continue to provide these services for the foreseeable future. Mr Thomas had been campaigning in Mount V's favour, but the news he was relaying did not seem to be hopeful:

Dear Graham,

I understand Watford General and Hillingdon Hospital are the most likely sites for the Mount Vernon Cancer Centre but none of this is confirmed or locked down. There is still the very outside possibility of it staying put or moving to another site, but Watford or Hillingdon appear most likely at the moment.

That sounded a gloomy prognosis, I feared. Yes, of course, people would still be able to access treatment, and probably many of the same staff would be able to move with the Cancer Centre, but inevitably, some of them would not be able to, or wouldn't fancy the new arrangement. And however well-equipped a new location was, it would take time to build a team-spirit amongst those who worked there and for patients used to one kind of experience to react to a new one – even though one might hope that in terms of facilities it would be just as good as, or even better than, Mount V.

I confess that as a result of my own experiences I was biased towards the thought that money should be spent on upgrading Mount V, rather than starting completely again elsewhere. In October 2021, Gareth Thomas' website was campaigning that 'the Government should be investing in Mount Vernon, not threatening it with closure.'

Remarkable goings-on overnight from 15 to 16 March, as we began to hear, via a WhatsApp group, of a couple of South African-variant Covid cases detected in our area. We may be contacted to take tests. There was also a video message on my phone from MP Gareth Thomas, also warning that we may have to be tested.

When I went out for the papers in the morning, I walked back via the local testing centre and volunteered myself to be 'done'. They asked for my postcode and consulted their pieces of paper. One chap said, 'Go in and be tested.' His boss said, 'No, we don't have his postcode written down.'

I walked away, frustrated, and as I turned a corner away from where the tests were happening, it was to see on a small building right in front of me, in large, red, capital letters on a white background, the word: 'SHARPE'.

I walked past, a little spooked (it transpired that the sign was promoting a new dance school), and when I got home, wrote up my experiences for my Facebook followers, posted alongside the SHARPE photograph, still none the wiser about whether I would end up having to be tested...

A day or two later, Sheila and I, along with the rest of our street, received a late-night leaflet through the door, shouting at us in black and red capital letters that: 'THE SOUTH AFRICAN VARIANT OF COVID HAS BEEN FOUND IN YOUR NEIGHBOURHOOD'.

Calming down, into a combination of upper and lower case, it went on to explain: 'We're asking everyone who receives this flyer to take part in testing. This is to check whether the variant is present in the community.' From the logos on the leaflet, I judged that 'we' meant Harrow Council, NHS Test and Trace and KEEP HARROW SAFE.

Fair enough. So, we logged on to the given place and were able to book tests at the local Arts Centre, a five-minute walk away – yes, to the one which had just turned me down because they didn't have my postcode logged, but let's not beat them up about that – for the very next morning.

It transpired that we needed both a lateral and a PCR test, whatever they may have been – the first one giving a result within an hour and the second taking a couple of days. The people administering the tests were, as ever, friendly, helpful and accommodating, so the process did not take long.

Fortunately, we returned negative results for both tests, and so did everyone else in our local WhatsApp group, which was encouraging.

A message arrived that evening from PC UK:

How do you feel about lockdown lifting, Graham?

We can't wait to see supporters like you face-to-face when we get back to matches, marches and making new friends across the country.

To make sure you get the best possible experience and feel safe, we'd love to know more about the kinds of events you'd feel comfortable attending in the coming months.

Please take this quick survey to help us understand how you feel about lockdown restrictions lifting.'

Odd? What had this got to do with working against PC, I wondered. Oh, well, so I'd do them a favour and take the survey, which they assured me wouldn't take longer than five minutes to complete... Most of the questions seemed to be designed to find out what PC UK fundraising events would be of appeal after lockdown restrictions were lifted... This was one of them: 'Could Prostate Cancer UK do anything to make you feel more confident about participating in our in-person events in the coming year? (Please select all that apply)'.

I ticked the box for a 'guaranteed refund', as there wasn't an answer saying: 'It doesn't matter, I won't be participating in such events in any case.' It took me seven minutes to fill it in, but it left me with a worrying feeling that it was all about how best they could raise money, rather than about anything aimed at directly helping the likes of me.

On 22 March, I read that PC UK had claimed that '8,600 fewer men started treatment' from April 2020 to January 2021, with the charity's chief executive Angela Culhane quoted as saying: 'Many more men could be diagnosed when it is too late for them to be cured.'

A new device which apparently 'sniffs out chemicals in breath' could be used 'to identify people with colon cancer, tuberculosis, prostate cancer, bladder cancer, regional pain syndrome and epilepsy', by identifying patterns of volatile organic compounds in bodies, reported the *Daily Mail* on 23 March 2021.

Its sister paper, the *Mail on Sunday*, had two days earlier written about early research into 'a new breed of drugs' known as antibody drug conjugates (ADCs), for which 'trials [were] under way to test the effectiveness of the experimental therapy on breast and prostate cancer'. This treatment was, reported the *Mail*, 'highly accurate. Targeting tumours without harming healthy tissue.'

It's the morning of 25 March 2021, I'd brought our morning cups of coffee (Sheila) and tea (guess) in. Sheila was reading the latest edition of *Woman & Home* magazine, which she handed wordlessly to me, pointing to a two-page spread. It was headlined 'Prostate Cancer BE AWARE' and was put together by clinical nurse specialist in prostate cancer, Karen Walker, and Saheed Rashid, MD of BXTAccelyon, 'leading providers of brachytherapy', who, I read, 'explain what women need to know'. A subheading asked: 'Could you help spot the symptoms and save a loved one's life?'

It was an interesting read with short sections headed: 'What is the prostate?', 'Prostate problems', 'What symptoms should I look out for?', 'Getting Diagnosed' and 'What if it turns out to be cancer?'. Ms Walker advised: 'Many people think it's a death sentence if they're diagnosed with metastatic prostate cancer. But it very often isn't, and many men may live with it for several years with the right treatment.'

Mr Rashid wrote: 'The most common early signs include difficulty starting urination, weak or interrupted flow of urine, the need to urinate more often, difficulty emptying the bladder completely, pain or burning during urination and loss of bladder control.' He reminded readers that 'there's a high chance these symptoms could be caused by conditions other than prostate cancer.'

The accompanying editorial was well written, informative and certainly not over dramatic, but found the right balance between alarming and reassuring possible sufferers...

35

IN WHICH MY MP GETS IN TOUCH

FRIDAY, 26 MARCH 2021 was a sad day – the day when I finally had to admit that my tub of Sudocrem antiseptic healing cream, given to me by an angel of mercy in nurse's garb some years ago, was finally and irrevocably, to the point where I'd had to buy another... empty. This soothing balm had protected, restored and caressed some of my more private areas of skin during its various trials and tribulations and I would happily admit to being addicted to the stuff, almost certainly for the remainder of my time on this mortal coil.

Taking my mind off Sudocrem, though, an email-cum-letter arrived from my MP, David Simmonds, to whom I had written about the uncertain future facing Mount V and, inevitably, the great staff I had met during my time being treated there.

Dear Graham,

Thank you for getting in touch to share your concerns about the future of the Cancer Centre.

I recently met with the team at NHS England who are leading on this project and I do understand the issues which are at play. There was previously a clinician-led review of the site, and they made a number of recommendations for how the cancer centre needs to be running going forward.

The first of these was a change in admissions policy. The reason for this is that far too many patients were being admitted and then later requiring transfer to another site. This admissions policy has now been changed but it does expose some of the other long-term problems.

The second recommendation was that the cancer centre needs to be run by a specialist cancer trust and not a general hospital trust. This is now in the process of taking place and from next year the site will no longer be run by East and North Hertfordshire NHS Trust and will transfer to UCLH [University College Hospitals]. This will not affect the on-the-ground staffing as the clinical team will remain the same, it is just a change of management with better specialism.

The final and most significant change is connected to the first point and that is that the Centre needs to be located on an acute site. The reason for this is because as populations are getting older, more patients are also living with other illnesses or conditions which require treatment alongside their cancer treatment. Furthermore, when complications arise from these therapies, patients require acute clinical opinions from other specialties. This cannot be provided for at Mount Vernon and so hence the need for a new site.

The NHS have been open about the options this presents.

The first option is a complete move to a new acute site and the second is a majority move with a smaller day centre remaining. This second option is obviously the best-case scenario from our point of view and is the option I have now been pushing for. At present this is the preferred option within the NHS.

In terms of the move, the emerging option which looks to be most suitable is to have the centre located at Watford. This centre would be a standalone centre, within its own building and would continue to be run by UCLH. However, it would offer an enhanced service from what it is currently able to offer. Some of the sickest patients are currently having to travel into London because of the limitations of the existing site and facilities.

I will be honest with the fact that the most affected patients are going to be those living in Hillingdon. However, given the size of the Mount Vernon catchment area, and that only 14% of their patients are from Hillingdon, we need to be realistic about where the most appropriate site might be. The team on this review have done a lot of research on travel times to all of the possible options and that is why Watford is appearing to be the preferred option. Given all this context, I think the most effective thing to do is to ensure we retain the day centre as has been discussed.

I am continuing to follow this all closely and a full public consultation is due to launch in June this year ahead of a final decision being made in October but this is where my thoughts are currently at.

Best wishes,

David

David Simmonds CBE MP
Member of Parliament for Ruislip, Northwood and Pinner

I was not sure whether this was good or bad news, and would have to read it through again and compare it with what I had heard from Gareth Thomas, to make my mind up.

A day later, I had a lengthy chat on the phone with Ron, who was feeling a little down following a recent family bereavement. I liked to think that we both felt a little more cheerful after our conversation, which encompassed many matters of relevance for both of us. The question came up, of how it was that though I had stopped having my three-monthly Zoladex injections, I still seemed to be experiencing a number of hot flushes. Did they gradually die off (or do I?) or was there some other effect at work? I must ask Dr A at our next appointment, I thought, if I'm still getting them.

Seeking a little more info, I had a look at what Cancer Research UK had to say on the subject:

Hormones occur naturally in your body. They control the growth and activity of normal cells. Testosterone is a male hormone mainly made by the testicles.

Prostate cancer usually depends on testosterone to grow. Hormone therapy blocks or lowers the amount of testosterone in the body. This can lower the risk of an early prostate cancer coming back when you have it with other treatments. Or it can shrink an advanced prostate cancer or slow its growth.

Low levels of oestrogen can cause low levels of the hormone norepinephrine. This hormone helps your body to regulate temperature. Low levels of norepinephrine may lead to increases in core body temperature. This can cause hot flushes in women going through the menopause.

Doctors think this might be the same reason that men get hot flushes when they have hormone therapy.

Some treatments such as goserelin (Zoladex) cause hot flushes in most men. Treatments called anti-androgen drugs are less likely to cause hot flushes. An example of an anti-androgen is bicalutamide.

For many people, hot flushes gradually get better over several months. For some people the flushes last as long as they are having treatment. They do tend to happen less often over time.

Hmm. I wasn't clear about how quickly they might stop after Zoladex was discontinued. Reading up about the Zoladex implants I had had for two years, I learned:

Common side effects

These side effects happen in more than 10 in 100 people (10%). You might have one or more of them. They include:

Hot flushes and sweats

We have some tips for <u>coping with hot flushes</u> and the possible treatments for men and women. Talk to your doctor if your hot flushes are hard to cope with. They might be able to prescribe you some medicines.

Then... I found this: 'This can continue for some time after you stop having goserelin.' 'Some time', then. I didn't like to ask, but how long was some time, would you think?

Wandering hopelessly around the pages of the PC UK website, failing yet again to find the page on which I was supposed to be logging my 11,000 steps or more each day, although for the past two or three times I had actually managed to locate it, I had been unable to add my steps due to some malfunction.

This time I stumbled across this notice:

We'll be transparent about the use of your donations.

You can see regular updates on how we spend your donations, and read all about how your support helps in our annual report.

65p in every £1 is spent directly on our objectives (2019-20 figures). We invested the rest in fundraising and the efficient running of the organisation.

So, there it was. Over one third of the money raised by donors goes to meet operational costs.

I couldn't find similar figures on the Cancer Research UK website, but there was this, dated April 2020:

Our CEO, Michelle Mitchell, was paid £244,000 between April 2019 and March 2020.

Cancer Research UK employs nearly 4,100 staff around the UK in a wide range of roles, including to raise funds and to carry out cutting-edge research. This is a complex organisation to lead.

We also supported the work of more than 4,000 scientists, technicians and other cancer research staff throughout the UK with research grants between April 2019 and March 2020.

Cancer Research UK is the world's leading charity dedicated to saving lives through research. We've been at the heart of the progress that has already seen survival in the UK double in the last 40 years. Every step we make towards beating cancer relies on vital donations from the public.

We promise to spend your donations wisely. We aim to make sure that at least 80p in each £ we receive from donations is available to help beat cancer.

We employ people who make a real difference and will help us achieve our ambition of seeing 3 in 4 people surviving their cancer by 2034.

Another section revealed that:

We expect our income to fall by at least 20-25% in the next financial year as a direct result of this pandemic.

We fund approximately 50% of all cancer research in the UK. To ensure we can continue to have this role in the long term, we need to shore up our income in the short term. We're reducing our operational costs as much as possible and freezing recruitment. Our Executive Board has taken a 20% pay cut and we're entering consultation with our staff to apply a similar reduction to their salaries and enrol a substantial number of people onto the government's new furlough scheme. It's likely that we'll have to make more difficult decisions over the coming weeks and months.

Unfortunately, these steps are not enough for us to confidently protect our future. With great regret, we've also had to take immediate action to reduce our spending on research funding. Our institutes' and existing response-mode funding will be cut by 5-10% and our centres and wider infrastructure by up to 20% this year. These cuts are substantial and will set back the cancer research effort within the UK, potentially for many years. We've also taken the decision to postpone any new funding commitments, which means no new research projects will be funded for at least the first half of this year.

36

IN WHICH I FILL IN ANOTHER SURVEY

IDLY LOOKING around on the internet, I found an invitation to take part in a survey for people with, or who have had, PC, so I took it. I'm still not sure who the organisers are, but I saw no downside to answering the questions, which I duly did. Here's the introduction I received:

Welcome – and thank you for your interest. This is a scientific project – your contribution is extremely important.

Through taking part you may be helping to ensure improved understanding of the needs and experiences of people with prostate cancer.

One of the questions I answered, was one which I had raised very much earlier in the treatment process I went through. It read: 'I would like a central source on the internet that contains up to date and complete information about cancer.' The answers varied, depending on how keen the respondent was to see such a thing and I signed up to the highest level of interest in so doing. How it would be achieved and financed were really not my concerns to worry about, but I believed a sponsor would not be difficult to acquire and that once up and running, organisations and people involved would want to be seen to be featuring on the site.

The next morning I received a follow-up email:

You are receiving this email because you participated in our prostate cancer survey. Thank you again for that!

Where are we at the moment?

So far, almost 5,000 people have taken the survey – great! Thanks to all who invested time in it! The interest is the same in all three countries (Germany, USA and UK) – so we will have enough information to compare the experiences of patients in these three countries.

What's next?

The survey remains open to participants until 15,000 complete questionnaires have been collected. That will be the case in mid-April. After that, the data will be compared for evaluation and subjected to a variety of statistical analyses.

When are results expected?

The results are expected in June. It is planned to present the results in a scientific publication. Participants who have provided their contact details, as you have, will also receive information about this. Until then, we will contact you from time to time and report on the progress.

Best regards,

CIURO

Not only did I receive this follow-up, but my publisher also sent me an email asking whether I'd seen this 'interesting survey' which had popped up on his own Facebook timeline – which was, of course, this very one. How or why it had arrived on his page, we have no idea.

I wondered whether, and when, we might hear any details of the results of this survey...

37

IN WHICH I AM LESS-THAN-SYMPATHETIC TO A SCRUFFY LOOKING CHAP

WEDNESDAY, 31 March 2021 – the final day of my participation in the PC UK 11,000 steps per day in March fund- and awareness-raiser.

Wednesday had become 'Waitrose day' during the pandemic. So the only opportunity to get in some early steps was after arriving in the Waitrose car park at just after 9am, and completing a few circuits as Sheila bustled about searching for a germ-free trolley in which to stash the mysterious cleaning stuffs to which she seems addicted.

On my first time round, I noticed a scruffy-looking chap, crouching on the ground, looking, forgive me for my knee-jerk reaction, like a 'homeless beggar'. A shopper was approaching him and beginning to engage him in conversation. On my second circuit, the two were still conversing, as a lady clad in supermarket-branded clothing approached, looking somewhat less friendly than the male shopper. She was reminding the scruff that he had been removed from the area on numerous occasions and would shortly be asked to leave again, asap. He did not appear overly concerned by this information, and his friendly shopper pal was arguing on his behalf.

As I returned on my third circuit the scruff had scarpered, the shopper and the shop assistant likewise. This might have been the same person already responsible for verbally abusing my wife when she had declined the request to contribute to his financial wellbeing, with my 100 per cent backing.

As we later drove out of the Waitrose car park to return home, I nearly ran the scruff over – not intentionally on this occasion – as he went back to resume his trade.

I duly completed the 11,000 steps a day challenge – and not only that, I even added 14 additional steps to the minimum number just to finish in style. When I tried to register this number with the website, it was having nothing to do with it, and I admitted defeat and gave up – at least I hadn't done that during the actual walking.

When I was approaching the final stages of March Into March, I came up with an idea which might remove my major objection to charity promotions. Surely when donating money, it would make sense for the recipient to offer the donor the option of deciding for themselves what percentage of their gift should go to the actual research, and how much should be contributed towards the salaries of those working for the charity.

This would alleviate most of my misgivings about how open the various recipient charities are about what goes where, once they get their hands on the donations. I didn't imagine that most donors would be as curmudgeonly as me... Some would probably be quite happy to leave it to the individual charity to decide how much goes where. But those who *are* could then specify for themselves: 'I want 99% of this going directly to research – do what you like with the remainder.'

If this were to lead to charities pleading poverty to the powers-that-be and going cap in hand to the government for the money to pay their staff, then so be it. I do think the money for all research of this nature should come from a central amount determined by the government. Anyone wishing to pay more to the central amount would be able to do so by paying an additional sum from their weekly or monthly pay packet back to the authorities to be spread around to deserving good causes.

Okay, okay, I know – dream on.

On 1 April I saw an extremely emotive story appear in the media, about a leading brain surgeon calling for an inquiry into assisted dying which he described as 'absolutely essential'.

Seventy-one-year-old Henry Marsh, who had advanced prostate cancer, joined politicians pressing for a review into this perennially controversial issue. The retired neurosurgeon had received his cancer diagnosis six months earlier, and told the BBC: 'It is extraordinarily difficult to think about your own death. My own suspicion as to why the opponents to assisted dying oppose a public inquiry is they fear that actually the evidence is so strong that their hypothetical arguments against it don't hold water, that they will lose the debate.'

Fifty MPs and peers had written a joint letter to Robert Buckland, the then justice secretary, in which they demanded that assisted dying legislation be looked at again. The petition was led by Humanists UK and claims that the UK has fallen behind the rest of the world on assisted dying laws, and that parliament 'cannot turn a blind eye' to the issue. Mr Marsh said that being told he had terminal prostate cancer left him 'filled with dread' at the thought of dying slowly. The typical mortality rate for people in stages three and four of the disease is between one and five years. Assisting a suicide is a crime in England and Wales, punishable by up to 14 years in jail.

Speaking about his diagnosis, Mr Marsh, who was due to start radiotherapy treatment in a few months' time, told the BBC he was 'deeply shocked and terribly frightened and upset' as it 'gradually dawned on him how serious the situation was.' In the *Daily Mail*, he added: 'Having spent a lifetime operating on people with cancer, the prospect of dying slowly from it myself fills me with dread.' 'Despite the best efforts of palliative medicine, I know that dying from cancer can still be a very horrible business – for both patient and family, despite what the opponents of assisted dying claim.'

And I also received a request to sign a petition, headed: 'Stop unnecessary cancer and early deaths caused by the Covid disruption and save thousands of lives.' I read a little more: 'Experts are warning that as many as **35,000 cancer patients could die unnecessarily** as a result of the impact of the pandemic on cancer services.' Okay, a little vague but seemed to tie in with stuff I'd been reading.

It continued: 'Please sign this petition to urge Matt Hancock to boost cancer services, at all stages of the cancer pathway, to stop tens of thousands of cancer patients dying unnecessarily.' So I signed – why wouldn't I, really? There had already been 376,192 signatures appended, I learned. The petition was started by Craig and Mandy Russell, the parents of a 31-year-old bowel cancer victim:

This is my daughter Kelly, she died tragically aged 31 due to bowel cancer. Her loss has been devastating to our family. **Her life expectancy was drastically cut short after her chemotherapy stopped as a direct result of Covid.** Across the UK, people have had their cancer treatments impacted – so I've started this petition calling for the Government to take urgent action, before it's too late.

You may have seen our Kelly's story featured in a recent *Panorama* programme called 'Britain's Cancer Crisis' which showed the extent of the problem. Experts are warning that as many as **35,000 cancer patients could die unnecessarily** as a result of the impact of the pandemic on cancer services.

I have to say, though, I wasn't overly impressed, having added my name to the petition, to be hassled by Change.org to donate money, and to share the petition on various online platforms. I wasn't sure high-pressure salesmanship was the best look for a charity appeal.

And then they sent me another message: 'The petition still needs your help Graham... By signing your next petition – and another petition after that – you'll see how easy it is to bring about lasting change. Check out these petitions that need your support next.'

Come on, no. The petition I was interested in needed me to sign it, which I'd done. So now what? Don't start trying to virtue-shame me, for Heaven's sake... I thought. I was NOT going to 'check out' those petitions. Sorry.

38

IN WHICH I SURPRISE MYSELF BY TURNING DOWN A SECOND JAB!

I HAD a bizarre experience on the evening of Saturday, 3 April when, at just after 6pm, I had a call from the place where I'd had my first Covid jab – Barnet FC's ground, The Hive – asking if I'd like to come in for my second that very evening.

The trouble was, I had already booked the second for a fortnight's time, and I was happy and psychologically prepared for that date. I'd also have had to drop everything there and then, to get over there to be 'done' that evening, and was concerned that it might even be a little too early, as the recommendation was to have it between ten and 12 weeks after the first jab, and to have it at this point would put me just under the ten weeks.

Also, I'd already taken the trouble to walk up to the location I'd booked – the Grimsdyke Golf Club, about a 15-minute stroll away, compared with the half-hour drive to The Hive – to check out where I'd be going. It felt wrong at this stage to change locations, even though it would be returning to where I'd had the first.

However, I was then able to ask whether instead of me, my wife could be booked in for her second, which was duly done, so she would now be 'done' two days before I would, on the 15 April, and she'd have it at The Hive as she'd done the first time round.

The gentleman who made the phone call had hesitated before speaking when I answered, so I had instantly assumed that this was yet another of the regular two or three scam calls we'd been getting for the past couple of weeks. I'd almost slammed the phone down in a rage when no one answered my 'Hello'. That wouldn't have been a good move, as the chap then told me they'd had to make

900 calls that day to book people in, and he'd probably just have moved straight on to the next one on the list if the line had gone dead.

Naturally I now started having second thoughts. Should I just have accepted the initial invitation and legged it straight over to Barnet's ground? No point going through that mental debate, I soon realised. You've made your decision, so stick to it, and be happy with it!

Through the door, contained amongst some blurb-y leaflets included with a magazine to which I subscribe, came a small publication of 16 pages, entitled 'PROSTATE PROBLEMS? – Finally Solved!' I flipped through it, and in the centre spread found a double-page article assuring me in a headline that: 'The Turkish male population has virtually no prostate problems.'

I read on with interest: 'To understand why the level of prostate problems was so low in Turkey – it is the lowest in the world... Turkish men shared an ancestral dietary habit that protects them from prostate problems.' Of course, I understood that there was a difference between prostate 'problems' and 'cancer', but I was in no doubt that this leaflet was designed to confuse those reading it into assuming, that the one was very similar to the other.

So I googled the World Health Rankings where I read: 'According to the latest WHO data published in 2018 Prostate Cancer Deaths in Turkey reached 8,249 or 2.03% of total deaths. The age adjusted Death Rate is 27.22 per 100,000 of population ranks Turkey #39 in the world. [sic]' Which was not quite the 'lowest in the world'...

On page 5, I read that there were 'three prostate diseases' which were 'Prostatitis', 'Enlargement of the prostate' and 'Cancer of the prostate'.

On page 6 of this publication, I discovered that the traditional 'finger up the bum' method of checking the prostate was now 'all in the past!' and that there was 'A quick and reliable test that you carry out yourself!' to 'reveal if you have prostate problems'.

Want to know how? 'The arc of your urine changes shape if you have prostate problems. To check it, you need to measure, by placing a ruler at the end of your penis, the stream up to pinch point... generally located between 2 and 5cm after the end of the penis on the urine stream.'

With us so far? Simples, isn't the word, is it? And on pages 14, 15 and 16, the magic potential cure was outlined under a '100% SATISFACTION OR MONEYBACK GUARANTEED' offer. It's all to do with 'pomegranate polyphenols', by the way. I didn't order anything from them.

The *Mail on Sunday* for 4 April brought news of 'Treatments for cancer – in your own living room', reporting in a story by Jonathan Neal that NHS patients 'could' receive 'cutting-edge' treatments at home in order to avoid them having to undergo regular hospital visits. Reporting that 'up to 100,000 patients with breast, bowel, lung, prostate or melanoma skin cancer' could benefit, the story explained that those suitable could be given initial treatments in a clinic but may then be able to 'opt to have the rest of their treatments at home'. The patients would not be left to treat themselves – their drugs would arrive via a pharmacist and specialist nurses would visit to administer them.

This new system was already in operation via The Christie NHS Foundation Trust in Manchester and was to be rolled out more widely.

On the same day I was asked to sign a 'Keep Pinner shisha free' petition by Change.org. I did not.

6 April I was asked to sign a 'Dog on dog attack' petition by Change. org. I did not. Then I received an email from PC UK, telling me 'We'd love to get to know you better, Graham', which made me put my suspicious-hat on immediately:

Thank you for signing our letters to NICE and Janssen, Graham.

You've helped to make a potentially huge impact for men with newly diagnosed, high-risk advanced prostate cancer.

12,673 of you signed the letters to show you stand with men caught in the middle of their drug approval tug-of-war.

Here's what you've helped to change so far:

Our campaign hit press in early March, including the *Times*, the *Express* and the *Telegraph*, spreading our message wide and putting pressure on NICE and Janssen.

Janssen and NICE then answered one of our calls and agreed to a meeting.

NICE acknowledged our plea to use population-wide evidence. They contacted key stakeholders requesting more evidence on the benefit abiraterone can have for men who can't tolerate chemotherapy.

Our letters motivated NICE to work more closely with us on other treatments that could benefit these men too. We've been working hard to try to get these treatments approved.

This is all promising news. Thank you so much for your support. Our campaign continues...

We'll be part of further talks on abiraterone with NICE and Janssen this month and we'll keep you updated every step of the way. Look out for future emails to find out how you can continue the fight for better care for men everywhere.

This one I didn't mind having signed, and was pleased it might be having some positive effect.

39

IN WHICH I HEAR OF ANOTHER SAD LOSS TO PC

THE MAJORITY of my working life was quite closely involved with horse racing, and this was the main source of income for my company, William Hill, for most of my time there – about 90% of its turnover when I joined in the early '70s, but probably down by almost half, as betting turnover soared on other sports, due to live TV coverage, by the time I left in 2017. Over the years I met many people associated with the racing world. One of them, a legendary trainer called Martin Pipe, was a great help when I was writing a biography of the hugely wealthy, and hugely eccentric, racehorse owner and gambler Dorothy Paget.

Martin invited me down to his stables on a couple of occasions to allow me to look through his archive of material about, and once belonging to, Dorothy and we became friendly. So I was quite affected to read the letter he had written to the *Racing Post* about his relationship with a five-time English table tennis champion, who became his assistant:

We are all saddened by the death of our dear friend George 'Chester' Barnes, an instantly recognisable character from the sports of table tennis and racing.

Chester possessed an infectious, charismatic personality that never failed to intrigue or entertain.

We have so many stories we could tell of his incredible life – the places he would go, the people he had met and some of the antics he had been involved in on and off the table tennis table and the racecourse – but there simply would not be enough room.

Everyone knew Chester. Indeed, he was once flown into the middle of a jungle to teach Hollywood superstar Steve McQueen how to play table tennis. On another occasion he also played Inspector Clouseau himself, Peter Sellers, although we are not sure who won!

We were very envious of Chester when only a few years ago we were in our hospitality marquee at the Cheltenham Festival when Penny Lancaster came calling for him. She had come to find Chester as Penny's husband and rock legend Rod Stewart wanted to see him. Chester had owned a pub in the east end of London and Rod and The Faces would practise in his skittle alley.

Chester's wife Jane and son Lester are fundraising in his memory in support of Prostate Cancer UK.

If you would like to donate to this amazing cause, please click on the banner on the left-hand side of David's [Martin's trainer son] website: www.davidpipe.com.

I was sure I remembered, years ago, seeing a TV programme in which Chester, a world-ranked player, number one in England during the 60s and 70s, challenged people to play him at table tennis, using the best available equipment, with Chester using as his bat - a frying pan. Of course, he still won...

**

Mid-April brought an email about the ongoing discussions over the future of Mount V:

Dear Graham,

I am just getting in touch to let you know that the team at NHS England have now started the next phase of the Mount Vernon Cancer Services Review. Having completed a large number of community engagement events between January and March this year they are now moving to explore specific areas of concern that came out of the meetings. It shall take the format of a series of 'working groups' covering 11 subject areas and they are keen to hear from interested current and former patients, their carers and families.

Best wishes,

Tom

Thomas Haynes
Senior Parliamentary Assistant to David Simmonds CBE MP
Member of Parliament for Ruislip, Northwood and Pinner

Working Groups April & May 2021

As a part of the Mount Vernon Cancer Services Review, a series of more than 70 online engagement events have been held with patients, families, support groups and stakeholders between January and March 2021.

These events have identified some key areas of concern for patients and families in the design and location of a new Cancer Centre and how care is delivered.

The next phase of the engagement will be to explore these key areas in depth with groups of interested current and former patients, their carers and families.

Radiotherapy

How could a networked radiotherapy work for patients and where might it be located? Participants will examine radiotherapy activity to explore and comment on networked radiotherapy model options.

Care Closer to Home

Patients and carers will have the opportunity to share ideas about aspects of their care at Mount Vernon Cancer Centre they feel could have taken place closer to their homes, or concerns about providing more care more locally. We will collect stories about some of the experiences of patients, for example, in travelling to MVCC for blood tests.

Patient Records

Patients will be invited to share their experiences, good and bad, of how their records have been used throughout their experiences, and offer their thoughts on the key priorities for improvements.

Building Layout and Design

These workshops will examine for a patient and carer perspective, what considerations need to be made in designing the layout of key areas in the Cancer Centre, like the Chemotherapy, inpatient and quiet spaces.

Disabled Access and Experience

This group will explore the experiences of patients and carers with disabilities, particularly in relation to access to and on the site to provide critical insight that will shape the planning of new facilities. As part of this work we will collect and explore patient stories.

Learning Disabilities

This piece of work will examine the needs of patients and carers with Learning Disabilities and seek to understand how best to engage with them and hear their stories.

Patient Information

This group will look at what support and information patients find most helpful and the value that patient support facilities adds to a patient's treatment and recovery. Participants will have the opportunity to use their ideas and experiences to help develop plans for the future of these services.

Transport and Access

This group will discuss issues and ideas around patient transport, public transport and access, to support discussions with transport providers.

40

IN WHICH I WONDER HOW IT WOULD HAVE BEEN HAD MY PC BEEN DIAGNOSED DURING THE COVID ERA

THE *DAILY Mail* Comment column of Monday, 19 April 2021, really brought home to me how fortunate I was to have been dealing with my PC treatment before the coronavirus era kicked in.

Yes, I was still officially a patient, and there was no guarantee that my current situation would remain as it was, with the regular biannual liaisons with Dr A continuing until the time she would suggest that they were no longer necessary (and I very much hoped, but doubted, that day would dawn).

So it was a genuine concern to read that: 'With 4.7 million patients now waiting for treatment, NHS Providers believes it could take five years to clear the backlog.' The paper was actually referring to this statistic to push their own agenda that lockdown 'must end on schedule by June 21 – and never be allowed to happen again'.

The next day, in the same paper, an amazing headline caught my attention: 'Calculator that adds up risk of prostate cancer'. My first thought was – that's all well and good, but like any other calculator, presumably it was only as good as the information fed into it, and the accuracy of the person doing the inputting.

The article claimed that the new calculator, developed by researchers at Oxford University – whose findings have been published in the *British Journal of General Practice* – 'is more accurate than the existing PSA test'. It works via a formula combining the PSA with a number of other factors, including age, ethnicity, body mass index, social deprivation and family history. This was initially impressive until you think, well, GPs would surely have most of this information to hand about individuals, so they may be able to draw a conclusion without the calculator.

However, Professor Julia Hippisley-Cox reckoned that her tests showed the calculator finding 68.2 per cent of PC cases, compared with 43.9 from PSA tests.

Simon Grieveson of PC UK felt, quite reasonably, that 'this now [needed] to be tested in large-scale clinical trials... to determine whether this model could offer real clinical benefit'.

On 22 April, I was contacted and told:

Hello from the CIURO team!

You are receiving this email because you participated in our prostate cancer survey.

Thank you again for that!

The survey ended successfully!

More than 15,000 people completed Part 1 of the survey and almost 10,000 Part 2 – great! Thanks to everyone who invested time in this!

This is how the number of participants is divided:

The survey was completed:

- 82% by patients,
- 16% by relatives or friends
- 2% by caregivers.

Participation Rate

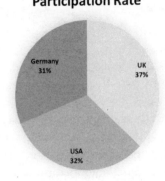

The average age is 70 years with participants' ages ranging from 44 to 98 – 'the Internet is only for the younger ones' seems not to be true!

What comes next?

The survey will now be evaluated. The immense amount of data (more than 10 million data points!) allows many different approaches and analysis models. We expect the first statements in June. Until then, we will contact you from time to time and report on the progress.

Best regards,

CIURO

Okay, I thought, fair enough – I was glad that I helped out, as this seemed to be a useful survey. Even though I didn't get any final results before the book went to press. However, the next petition I came across really didn't.

This is what I was asked to sign up to:

Since the 1970s it has been shown that 41% of all UK species (of bees) have declined. **The fact of the matter is heartbreaking**, so I have set about to see what local councils and individuals can do to make a difference.

Utrecht Council in Holland in 2019 have **transformed 316 bus stops into 'Bee Bus stops'.**

Installing green roof tops onto bus stops has created a bee friendly space for the endangered species. **The wildflower roof tops will also help absorb rainwater, capture dust or pollution from the air and regulate temperatures.**

In April 2020 in the UK, Cardiff Council in Wales introduced over ten bee bus stops with the same scheme.

I live in the city of Brighton and I believe they have at least 150 sheltered bus stops that could be put to great use by this project. I am currently counting the bus shelters in Brighton to get the exact number that could be used.

We *are* in an environmental crisis.

Kind regards,

Yazmin

Yazmin, I thought, you must bee joking. Anyway, much though I love the city, and frequently visit for the sheer buzz of the place and to rummage around in its record shops to hive off some desirable vinyl, I do not, and never will live in Beerighton, my honey.

41

IN WHICH I HEAR AN UNEXPECTED STORY FROM A WORK COLLEAGUE

'M' AND I had been work colleagues for a while. He left before I did. He used to live in the same town as me, but then moved away. We had kept in touch occasionally, mainly via Twitter.

One evening in late April 2021, he contacted me to let me know that Michael Portillo's latest television jaunt had been filmed in and around the town where I still lived, and was going to be screened that very evening. He just thought I might be interested, and how was I?

I told him that I had attended the same school as Mr Portillo, albeit a couple of years ahead of him. Our paths subsequently occasionally crossed because of his role on the judging panel for the Booker Prize, and again the time that I stumbled across a vaguely lost-looking Portillo wandering haphazardly along a well-known Central London thoroughfare, glancing into the windows of restaurants but looking unsure about his ultimate destination. I'd greeted him as a fellow 'Old Gayt', (we both attended Harrow County Grammar School, whose alumni are known as Old Gaytonians) and, after mentioning our Booker connection – I set the odds for bets on the outcome – our conversation was short and unmemorable.

We'd also once clashed at a press conference when he was chairing the Booker judging panel and I criticised the absence of a well-backed title from the just announced shortlist. I had wondered why it was missing. Michael won our little debate by pointing out that he had read more of the books entered than I had!

So, yes, I told M, I might be interested in watching Michael's programme, if only to see what bizarre colour combination of clothes he'd been kitted out in by 'wardrobe' on this occasion. I duly thanked my former colleague for letting me know, asking after his health – as you do – and he responded thus: 'On the personal front, it's been a terrible year. Won't bore you with all the details. Basically, had a cardiac arrest last May, and was in intensive care for four nights. Lucky to be alive. Also had prostate cancer – 20 radiotherapy sessions. But I'm still here, and trying to get back to tennis after an 11-month gap. Hope your health has been better than mine.'

This was shocking news and of course the PC reference made me want to know more. Here was the 'more' that came when I asked:

'I'll be 73 in May. I spent my 72nd birthday unconscious in intensive care. Did you have the hormone injections during your radiotherapy treatment? Three days after the first one I collapsed on the tennis court. I think that's what triggered the cardiac arrest, though of course I had diseased arteries, and now I have two stents. I'm only alive because a retired GP was playing on an adjacent court. He did mouth to mouth and CPR (breaking most of my ribs in the process) before the ambulance arrived. My wife knew nothing about it until police arrived on the doorstep. I'm now on eight tablets a day, seven of which are for life.'

Crikey. Could his PC treatment in general, or hormone injections specifically, have triggered his cardiac arrest? How alarming was it to read that?!

As for PC, it's very common isn't it? My treatment finished in October 2020. Hereford for 15 sessions, Cheltenham for five. My PSA in February 2021 was 0.08. I have another PSA in three weeks then a tele-con with the oncologist. I guess you didn't have to travel far for your treatment? Do you now have regular PSA tests?

The tennis is very low-key – social doubles. Have been trying to build my strength up with three or four long walks each week.

To me it was too much of a coincidence – the first exercise taken after the jab resulted in a near death experience. The GP disagreed with me, however the oncologist thought it was possibly related.

Not seen the doctor who saved me – in fact we've never met. My plan is to take him and his playing partner (who got the defibrillator going) out to lunch when permitted. The doctor is a member of the tennis club and it's likely I will meet him soon as he's listed for the social tennis. (I just started again last Friday.)

I think it's very good of you to write about your experiences, as ultimately it could save lives. Chaps I speak to about PC who've not been tested just tend to say 'I'm okay' or 'I don't have symptoms' (I didn't have any either). So any wider awareness will be welcome I'm sure. Willing to participate anonymously.

As for the future, here's my (optimistic) take. My PSA was 0.03 in October and 0.08 in February, so that's a growth of 0.05 in 3 months. Or 0.2 a year, so should take five years to go up to 1, if rate of increase were to be consistent.

May not be the case of course!

I haven't heard from M since.

The NHS was 'short of almost 2,000 radiologists needed to treat a growing backlog of patients' estimated the Royal College of Radiologists, according to a report in the *Times* on 28 April 2021. Then, a couple of days later, the *Metro* was telling me that 'a home test kit for prostate cancer could help diagnose aggressive forms of the disease early, while cutting hospital visits', explaining that for the trial '2,000 men in the UK, Europe and Canada' had been asked to send in two urine samples for laboratory analysis.

Other reports suggested that this potential system would make it easier for doctors to monitor 'low-risk' men being kept 'under surveillance' by doctors. Stressful hospital visits could be much reduced, said the reports, whilst such home tests 'may alert doctors to their cancer becoming more aggressive, using red-flag genetic changes in the prostate, which can be detected in the urine'.

The trial, targeting men usually aged between 55 and 80, had resulted from a 2019 study, that showed that urine tests can track 38 genes which can indicate whether men have aggressive PC and require urgent treatment.

PC charity Movember, which helped fund the trial, said they believed that the test had 'great potential to transform the way PC is managed'.

42

IN WHICH WATER IS TURNED INTO WHISKY

I WAS once at a very high-profile horse racing awards function, and, heading for the bar to get a round in, I found myself next to a chap I recognised, and identified as well-known wealthy racehorse owner, and former bookmaker, JP McManus.

He was just ahead of me in the queue and asked the barman for 'two sparkling waters, please'.

'Sorry, sir, we're out of bottles of water.'

Without any hesitation or deviation, McManus immediately said, 'Two large scotches, then, please.'

I looked at him, impressed, and gave a slight smile, receiving back a quick nod of the head. I didn't know until some while after that day, that JP, whose familiar green and yellow coloured hoops are well-known to almost all regular racegoers, was a fellow PC sufferer. He was diagnosed in 2009, and had successful treatment in America.

In a 2010 interview with Brough Scott in the *Racing Post*, almost a year to the day since JP, as he is affectionately called by virtually everyone in the racing business, had been diagnosed with PC, he observed: 'You know, a lot of good came out of the cancer. You see things in a different light. I got more out of it than I lost, and there was never a day I thought I wouldn't make it. It was caught at a very early stage. It wasn't all bad, it's an inconvenience – that's what it was.' Couldn't have put it better myself, JP...

Then I read a story in *The Sun*, revealing that another racing figure who had suffered from cancer, 1981 Grand National-winning jockey Bob Champion, now 72 years old, was apparently facing another health setback.

Bob, the article reported, was undertaking a charity walk to mark the number of days from his testicular cancer diagnosis on 24 July 1979, to when he received the all-clear on 31 January 1980.

Champion had thus far raised more than £55,000 on the walk, while his charity, The Bob Champion Cancer Trust, established in 1983, had raised millions over the years, and had helped fund research into PC (as previously mentioned in these pages).

However, the story explained that 'the ex-jockey [was] set to need treatment after doctors discovered a growth'. He was quoted as saying: 'I had a very bad back pain just before I started my walk and scans showed I have a tumour on my kidney which needs removing. I was determined I would carry on with my 40th anniversary walk though, as to raise money for the Bob Champion Cancer Trust has been my life's work and I didn't intend to fall at the final fence.'

I also received an update from Mike Cattermole (racing journalist/broadcaster, who is closely involved with the BCCT) in late August 2021, about four projects that the Bob Champion Cancer Trust had supported recently.

The Institute of Cancer Research had expressed gratitude to the BCCT 'for their generous support' for the collaborative project 'generating and exploiting massive volumes of data on the genetic and molecular characterisation of patients' prostate cancers. Using Big Data effectively will allow us to answer key questions in cancer research and treatment.'

The BCCT had been supporting the Prostate Urine Risk (PUR) project and as a result a home test kit had been developed. Professor Colin Cooper, who had dedicated much of his working life to researching PC, had been deeply involved in the PUR project launch, being trialled in the UK, Europe and Canada, also backed by Movember and PC UK.

He had developed a test to analyse historic biopsy samples of PC to identify a dangerous group of cancers known as 'tiger' cancers. 'Without the generous support of donors, none of these advances would have been possible,' said the professor, who believed they would help many patients to 'avoid unnecessary treatments which can carry associated side effects.'

***

One day, quite recently, I was having a shower when I suddenly spotted myself in the mirror of the wall cabinet, in which dwell such items as aftershave, Germolene, plasters, deodorant, Gengigel, razor blades and such like. I looked at my chest. Was I growing breasts? I'd heard and read that this could be a side effect of hormone treatment. Or was lockdown, during which I have to admit I'd probably been eating rather more than normal, albeit with the effects offset by increased activity, just making me a little fatter?

I consulted the Cancer Research UK website:

The adrenal glands produce a small amount of oestrogen in men. Hormonal treatments lower your testosterone and this changes the balance of hormones in your body. When oestrogen becomes higher, compared to the amount of testosterone, breast tissue can develop. Oestrogen stimulates the growth of breast tissue.

Breast swelling in men is gynaecomastia (pronounced guy-nee-co-mass-tee-ah).

Swelling can happen in either breast, or both breasts. It may be painful. It starts as fatty tissue. But it can develop into thicker (dense) tissue. This is glandular tissue.

I'd better keep an eye on this, I thought...

43

IN WHICH POSSIBLE PC PANDEMIC PANIC POINTED OUT

BRITAIN WAS at risk of 'replacing the Covid crisis with a cancer crisis', experts had said, reported the *Telegraph* on 24 May 2021. 'Official statistics show that more than 300,000 people have missed urgent checks for suspected cancer since the start of the pandemic.'

Cancer Research UK analysis indicated almost 40,000 fewer patients had begun cancer treatment during this time, a drop of 12 per cent. The charity warned that Britain was in danger of walking into a cancer crisis.

Newly diagnosed cancer patients were being reduced to speaking to specialists by phone or video call, rather than face-to-face, experts warned at the beginning of June 2021. The proportion of those told that they had PC but who then did not get an in-person consultation, had risen eightfold during the pandemic.

A survey by Prostate Cancer Research (PCR) revealed that patients feared important aspects of their condition might be missed. The new survey also showed that 65 per cent of UK PC patients believed cancer care had been compromised by the pandemic.

Around the same time, I also read that: 'A study of more than 6.3m men found that their risk of late-stage or fatal prostate cancer was significantly higher when at least one close family member had previously been diagnosed .'

***

I'd popped into a local Coral betting shop to check out if and how the environment in their branches had changed, now that they were allowed customers again after a lengthy lockdown layoff, which had been pushing punters towards online betting. Having spent over 40 years working in the bookmaking business, I had obviously retained an interest in what was going on in it, and I do enjoy the odd flutter now and then.

Perusing the racecards displayed on the shelves I noticed that there was an evening meeting at Sandown, so decided to make a small investment so that I could watch the races live on the TV later on, with a financial interest in the outcome. I then noticed that all of the races at Sandown appeared to be sponsored by the bookmaker whose shop I was standing in, and that one of them, the final race of the evening, was bizarrely called the 'Coral Supporting Prostate Cancer Handicap'.

Interesting, I thought, and looked at the rest of the race names to see whether this was perhaps an evening's racing devoted to the cause of supporting PC treatments. But there was no mention in any of the other race names of PC – one was even worryingly entitled the 'Beaten by a Length' race. Beaten by what implement was not explained.

It then struck me that in actual fact, calling a race 'Supporting Prostate Cancer' rather suggested that it was the disease being 'supported', rather than its victims. At the very least this was an insensitive title. Hadn't anyone checked or proofread any of the race details before approving them, I wondered? Maybe the paper I was reading this in had mistitled the race. I checked other papers and online racecards. No, 'Supporting Prostate Cancer' it was – everywhere.

Was this worth getting upset about? Possibly not to the majority of casual observers. But to me and very probably, many other PC sufferers, yes.

First of all, I checked the company's official website to see whether there might be any official awareness of this mistake, and/or some PC-treatment related material. I couldn't find anything PC-related on their site at all.

I contacted a good friend in the betting industry, who just happened to work in a senior position for Coral:

Popped into your branch in Hatch End this morning to check out what betting shops look like this side of the recent lockdown. I had a look at the card for this evening's Sandown meeting at which you sponsor all of the races.

The last race, the 8.30, caught my eye – 'Coral "Supporting Prostate Cancer" Handicap'. It caught my eye because I happen to have PC and I am currently writing a book about my experiences with it. It just struck me as a little odd that the race is called 'Supporting Prostate Cancer'.

Shouldn't it be 'Let's Beat Prostate Cancer' or something similar like 'Supporting Prostate Cancer Research' – the current name suggests that Coral are in favour of PC which I very much doubt is the case.

I have no wish to be churlish, but I then checked the Coral and Entain websites and could find no mention of any PC-related campaign going on, so I'm now baffled as to why this one oddly titled race is so named, or have I missed a whole campaign which it is part of? If so, I apologise...

There was no response whatsoever, initially. I waited patiently – unlike me, I know – before sending a reminder, which finally resulted in this brief response: 'Hi Graham, sorry I meant to reply. Yes, the race title was missing the letters "UK"... Prostate Cancer UK is Coral's company charity and we are raising money in our retail shops through staff fundraising activities and centrally organised events over the year.'

Okay, I was very pleased to hear that the company were raising money in their shops, although there was no indication whatsoever of any organised campaign in the branch I had visited.

I delved back into Google, inserting the phrase 'Prostate Cancer UK Coral bookmakers' and, to be fair, up came a November 2019 story:

Partnership aims to raise funds and increase awareness

A new charity partnership between the leading bookmaker Coral and Prostate Cancer UK, the largest men's health charity in the UK, kicks off this month with the twin aims of raising vital funds and increasing awareness of the risks of the most common cancer in men.

The three-year partnership was the result of a vote by Coral staff to choose a company-wide charity partner, and will see staff in Coral shops across the UK and at their London headquarters carry out a wide range of fundraising activities to champion Prostate Cancer UK's work of profiling the disease, as well as raise awareness of the risk of prostate cancer among Coral staff and customers.

I found some more positive info on the PC UK site:

Following a vote by Coral staff, Prostate Cancer UK and Coral will work together for three years (October 2019-October 2022) to form a charity partnership focused on increasing awareness of prostate cancer and its risks amongst Coral employees and customers.

Staff in Coral shops across the UK and at their London headquarters will also carry out a wide range of fundraising activities, including the sale of our Man of Men pin badge.

Right, now I'd go and see whether I could buy one of the pin badges in the local Coral branch.

Excellent, I could!

Still on the racing theme, I was watching the TV coverage from the 2021 Royal Ascot meeting on ITV when I was momentarily distracted. Feeling disgruntled, as my selections trundled along at the rear of each race, I then heard that a number of major bookmakers had announced that they would be donating their profits from the bets placed on the Britannia Stakes, on Thursday, 17 June, to a number of charities, amongst which was Prostate Cancer UK. It was later announced that over £1,000,000 was being distributed as a result of this not ungenerous gesture. At last, some positive news about something to do with the industry in which I was employed for most of my working life.

Bill Barber wrote in the *Racing Post* that:

A seven-figure sum is set to be split between a number of UK charities following a Royal Ascot fundraiser organised by the Betting and Gaming Council (BGC).

Prostate Cancer UK, Marie Curie, three Armed Forces charities and Care Radio will receive a share of £1.25 million from the profits made by participating bookmakers following Perotto's 18-1 success in the Britannia Stakes last Thursday.

44

IN WHICH BOB DYLAN PAYS TRIBUTE TO A GREAT CRICKETER

I WAS thinking of Bob Willis's wife, Lauren, as I read the following story: 'The England and Wales Cricket Board has decided to go blue at Edgbaston for the One Day International between England and Pakistan on the 13th of July to honour the legendary Bob Willis who died of prostate cancer in December 2019.'

Another report revealed:

Lauren Clark, the wife of the late Bob Willis, explains how the Bob

Willis Fund was established and how it hopes to help fight prostate cancer.

Edgbaston will turn #BlueForBob during England's final ODI against Pakistan on Tuesday to remember the late, great Bob Willis and raise awareness of prostate cancer research.

Willis – who took 325 Test wickets for England, including eight in that iconic Ashes spell at Headingley in July 1981, before becoming an acerbic, knowledgeable and revered Sky Sports pundit – passed away from prostate cancer in December 2019 at the age of 70.

Spectators are being urged to wear blue clothing to Tuesday's match to show their support for The Bob Willis Fund, co-founded by Bob's wife Lauren Clark and his brother David Willis.

The fund aims to support critical research into prostate cancer with the hope that a nationally accessible and accurate screening programme for the disease can be established and save lives.

Lauren – who had been so helpful as she assisted me in explaining the frustrating story of Bob's death from PC, and who had revealed how determined she was that something positive should emerge from it (in terms of preventing others from following his fatal course) – told me after the event that: 'The charity has been renamed The Bob Willis Fund [BWF], not Foundation, and we raised more than £300k at "Blue For Bob" day at Edgbaston. Bob's brother, David, and I are now working for the Bob Willis Fund, which is raising money and awareness for prostate cancer. We are also working closely with PC UK, but want to focus on the BWF.'

Lauren also told me how proud Bob would have been to know that his absolute musical hero, Bob Dylan, had agreed to become the Honorary Patron of the Fund. Dylan said: 'Bob Willis was a great sportsman who left too soon. I'm happy to help keep his flame and cause alive.' Another great friend of Bob Willis, Sir Tim Rice, is now the patron of the BWF.

Not as proud as he would be to know what fantastic work Lauren had done to keep Bob's memory and legacy alive in such a positive way, which would undoubtedly help many men to survive PC.

An article in the summer 2021 edition of my local *Hatch End Bulletin* brought an update from MP David Simmonds about the future of the Mount Vernon Cancer Centre:

The Cancer Centre needs to be run by a specialist cancer trust and not a general hospital trust... and from next year the site... will transfer to University College London Hospitals... the clinical team will remain the same... the Centre needs to be located on an acute site... because as populations are getting older, more patients are also living with other illnesses... which require treatment alongside their cancer... when complications arise from these therapies patients require acute clinical opinions from other specialties [sic]. This cannot be provided for at Mount Vernon.

The first option is a complete move to a new acute site and the second is a majority move with a smaller day centre remaining... This second option is obviously the best-case scenario from our point of view and is the option I have been pushing for.

He went on to explain that 'the most suitable' option was 'to have the centre located at Watford... a stand-alone centre within its own building,' which 'would offer an enhanced service from what it [was] currently able to offer'.

On Friday, 2 July 2021, the *Daily Mail* brought this news: 'a drug typically used to treat prostate cancer could help Covid patients, as it "significantly" reduces virus entry into the lungs, a study (led by the University of Essex) has found.' The drug treatment is called enzalutamide, which blocks the effect of testosterone on PC cell growth but which had now reportedly been discovered to block a protein that coronavirus uses to access lung cells'.

More positive information on 4 July, as a *Mail on Sunday* headline roared: 'Twin blasts that rein in terminal prostate cancer'. The story elaborated that: 'Men with incurable prostate cancer could be thrown a lifeline by a new approach that "doubles up" radiotherapy treatments.'

One 68-year-old patient in a trial, wrote Ethan Ennals, had been given six months to live but was still alive five years on after taking part in a trial of the new treatment, which involves immediately offering patients whose PC has spread to their bones, two specialist forms of radiotherapy – volumetric modulated arc therapy, and radium 223 – alongside hormone therapy.

'While it is by no means a cure, we are showing progress in extending the lives of patients,' said Professor Joe O'Sullivan, a specialist in radiation oncology at Queen's University, Belfast.

The *Telegraph* reported this on 7 July 2021:

The NHS is planning a £10 billion cancer blitz amid warnings from the Chief Medical Officer that the 'indirect effects' of the Covid pandemic are 'as major' as the crisis itself.

Sajid Javid, the Health Secretary, had vowed to 'bust the NHS backlog' saying he had been shocked to discover that around seven million people in need of help had not come forward during the pandemic.

There had been so many of this type of story of late, but one wondered whether it was just re-reporting of the same thing, or genuinely new initiatives to deal with the problems caused by Covid. We had to hope it was the latter, but could there have been a more cynical motive – to draw attention away from the stories showing that far fewer PC patients were being able to be diagnosed and/or treated during the pandemic?

A mere two days later and the *i* newspaper featured the headline

'New treatment for aggressive prostate cancer', over a story by Nina Massey, informing readers that those suffering from a 'particularly aggressive' form of PC could, research indicated, 'be treated more effectively by combining an existing targeted medicine with an experimental drug'.

The story explained that the combination included the hormone drug abiraterone and the new drug ipatasertib. Trials funded by Roche, across 200 sites in 26 countries and involving 1,101 patients, showed that this approach 'reduced the risk of death or cancer progression by 23 per cent compared with being treated by abiraterone alone'. Researchers were commencing 'a longer follow-up' in order to 'get regulatory approval or be accessed on the NHS'.

Once again, the human cost of PC was highlighted, when it was reported by the *Mail on Sunday*, on 10 July 2021, that award-winning disc jockey Jonathan 'Jono' Coleman 'had died at the age of 65 after fighting prostate cancer'. Born in London, but brought up in Australia, he was part of the popular 'Russ and Jono' duo, presenting shows on Virgin Radio in the 1990s. Once again, inappropriate cliches of 'fighting a battle' were wheeled out, probably without thought by the journalist reporting the sad death.

Shortly afterwards, I was reading the excellent 2021 book *Damage*, by my friend, and former *Boxing News* editor, Tris Dixon, in which he reports an interview he held with Leon Spinks, the boxer who, as little more than a rookie, caused a sensation by defeating the all-time Greatest, Muhammad Ali.

Leon had been through some hard times since and Tris had been to see him as part of his research for the book, which was about the forgotten, or ignored, virtual inevitability that being a boxer may well result in the participant suffering some form of brain damage or other major health problem in later life.

As if the interview with Spinks was not in itself heartbreaking enough, Tris closes it thus: 'Leon Spinks died around 18 months after my visit. He had prostate cancer and was 67.'

***

Two potentially dramatic boosts for PC patients were revealed in early September 2021, as, firstly, news broke in the *Daily Mail* that six major NHS hospitals were 'trialling the use of an algorithm which scans images of prostate biopsies to accurately detect cancer and determine how aggressive the disease is'. This could lead to a speeding up of both diagnosis and treatment, dramatically shortening the current processes.

The new algorithm, known as Galen Prostate, is reportedly 98% accurate in detecting PC, revealed a study published in *The Lancet*.

And Ethan Ennals of the *Mail on Sunday* reported that 'men with PC could soon be cured in less than two weeks thanks to a new high-speed radiotherapy technique – halving the time of standard treatment'.

The new approach would allow 20-dose treatments, which currently take a month to be given, to be delivered 'in just five big doses over seven to 14 days'.

Dr Alison Tree, study lead and consultant clinical oncologist at The Royal Marsden Hospital, told the paper that following trials with almost 900 patients: '[Their] data shows potentially curative prostate radiotherapy can be given with very few side effects for patients in a matter of days.' She added: 'I think there's a good argument for adopting it across the NHS.'

45

IN WHICH THE END MAY BE NOT-THAT-NIGH FOR MOUNT VERNON

ON 14 JULY 2021, I saw this on Facebook:

From 4 Aug 2021-10 Jan 2022, Prostate Cancer Research (PCR), in collaboration with Tackle Prostate Cancer, are bringing you a number of video webinars, hosted on Zoom, covering a diverse range of topics. These topics will be led by an expert(s) in their field discussing topics that our patient, partner, family and carer communities have told us they want more support and information on. All are welcome!

I was not sure I knew much about PCR so I took a look at their website, and ended up reading a very interesting section in which current 'unknowns' or 'unachievables' of PC treatment were being admitted and discussed:

What we still don't know about prostate cancer

Better understanding of prostate cancer will lead to new treatments, and using current treatments more effectively. Our review of peer-reviewed scientific papers identified the following gaps in our scientific knowledge of prostate cancer.

Underlying Biology

We need more understanding of the wider role of specific signalling pathways in prostate cancer and treatment resistance.

Treatment

We need to know more about why cancer spreads to bone and how to stop it, how to keep hormone therapy working for longer, and how to make immunotherapy work for prostate cancer.

Diagnosis

We need a more accurate test for prostate cancer, and more certainty about which prostate cancers need treatment and which do not.

Side Effects

Mitigating the harms caused by side effects of current prostate cancer treatment must be a priority.

The site showed a refreshing willingness to admit that there were gaps in knowledge and understanding of many matters related to PC...

What we are doing about knowledge gaps:

Some of our current projects are focusing on significant knowledge gaps. We also highlighted the knowledge gaps identified by this analysis as particular areas of interest in our 2020 grant call. Almost 40% of applications pertained to one or more of these areas, demonstrating that there are researchers with bright ideas willing to tackle these knowledge gaps, if funding is made available for them to do it. We will continue to monitor knowledge gaps and to adjust our approach where appropriate to meet them. Where prostate cancer shares a knowledge gap or unmet need with another disease, we will seek to develop a partnership to tackle it with other charities in that space. It is clear to us that charities could have much more impact if we worked together, and if we worked together with government.

'We've been forgotten, say patients with cancer' was the headline in the *Daily Mail* of 5 August 2021, the associated article reporting that cancer patients had been '"forgotten" during the pandemic with one in three suffering disruption to treatment'. The stat was taken from a Cancer Research UK survey of 900 patients, with 31% saying their care had 'deteriorated' compared with before Covid.

***

Having been a Luton Town supporter for over 60 years and a season ticket holder for many of those, I was already having an emotional day as I went back to Kenilworth Road on 7 August 2021. This was to see our opening home game of the Championship season against Peterborough, after well over a year's absence from the ground due to Covid restrictions.

We won the game 3-0 which was great, but it was just as heartening – no, moving – to hear and see the genuinely sympathetic – empathetic for many, I was sure – ovation the 10,000 capacity crowd gave on several occasions to the Hatters' iconic former player and current assistant manager Mick Harford, who had only relatively recently revealed he had PC.

'One Micky Harford, there's only one Micky Harford' was the chant swelling up three or four times during the game, causing one of the game's legendary 'hard' men to acknowledge the support from the predominantly male audience who were clearly aware of his recent revelation. One can only hope that those joining in with the chants would also ensure that they had themselves checked out as a result of the coverage surrounding Mick's situation.

While we were away on holiday in Jersey in mid-August 2021, I had my latest update from my oncologist, which showed that my PSA level had doubled since the previous one. As this meant that I was now at 0.02, up from 0.01, I wasn't unduly alarmed – nor was the oncologist herself, which was always reassuring. 'He is well and his PSA is satisfactory,' she wrote in the follow-up letter, confirming: 'He will have a further consultation in six months' time with a PSA prior.' Something to look forward to...

And the *Daily Mail* offered something else to look forward to, should it prove viable. The story in the paper on 12 August 2021 was headlined 'New hope for men suffering side effects of prostate ops', and began: 'Men who suffer erectile dysfunction after surgery for prostate cancer could benefit from shock-wave therapy.'

A British trial at Guy's Hospital was apparently seeking

participants: 'Treatment involves delivering a painless acoustic wave to the penis using a specialist probe for ten to 15 minutes. Volunteers will receive up to ten weekly sessions.' Okay, I thought, form an orderly queue...

This story prompted an anonymously authored piece in the *Telegraph* by a PC 'victim', suffering from erectile dysfunction as a result, in which he wrote: 'I didn't think that having ED would affect me but I was very wrong'. It's something that specialist nurse Sophie Smith often heard on the support helpline at Prostate Cancer UK. 'The side effects of treatment can be very impactful,' she told me, 'not just with radical prostatectomy but radiotherapy... and hormone therapy, too. A lot of the time, initially dealing with the cancer is at the forefront of your mind, and then it's that your waterworks are okay but erectile function gets pushed to the back of your mind until life moves on.

'Even if a man isn't sexually active, losing an erection is hugely impactful,' she continued. 'It's your manhood, your "maleness", what you've lived with forever... gone.'

At this point, I feel I should tell you that as a result of my own radiotherapy and three-monthly injection regime treatment, it was only in July 2021 that my wife and I resumed normal conjugal engagement. This happened on what used to be known as the 'honeymoon island' of Jersey, our resort of choice for summer hols for many years and where, perhaps, we are both much more relaxed and stress-free than is ever possible at home.

If I were being honest, I think I'd pretty much abandoned thoughts (hopes) that I'd ever experience such moments again. But I was so delighted when I did, that after several days I had to apologise to Sheila for becoming something of a sex junkie! Yes, yes, I know – *too* much information...

Cancer Research UK announced the following in August 2021: 'prostate cancer survival has tripled in the UK over the past 40 years – more than eight in ten patients are alive ten years after diagnosis – up from one in four in the 1970s'.

What I regarded as a counter-intuitive story emerged towards the end of August 2021, when a study of 400 men in the USA by Oakland University appeared to indicate that an enlarged prostate 'may protect men against developing prostate cancer'. The journal *The Prostate*, though, confessed: 'How an enlarged prostate could offer such protection is currently unclear.' This story coincided with hospitals and GPs in the UK being forced to cancel thousands – TENS of thousands, in fact – of blood tests, due to a severe global shortage of collection tubes, blamed on a combination of lack of raw materials, delays at borders and driver shortages.

The *Daily Mail*, still campaigning to raise awareness of PC and to improve treatment, revealed in September 2021, that: 'six major NHS hospitals are trialling the use of an algorithm which scans images of prostate biopsies to accurately detect cancer and determine how aggressive the disease is.' CEO of the technology arm of the health service, Matthew Gould, welcomed this news: 'We are currently caught between having too few pathologists and rising demand for biopsies. This technology could help and give thousands of men with prostate cancer faster, more accurate diagnoses.'

In a story revealing that 'a discount was agreed' for an 'effective and valuable' PC treatment, on 8 September 2021, it was explained in the *Daily Mail* that some 8,000 patients would now become eligible for treatment with apalutamide, also known as Erleada, which 'blocks the effect of testosterone on prostate cancer cells' – which sounds rather like what the Zoladex I'd had for a couple of years' treatment was used for.

'It is for those with hormone-related prostate cancer at high risk of spreading,' added the story. Oh yes – the cost of this treatment? Apparently a 'confidential discount' would reduce the price from the current £2,735 for a pack of 112, according to the National

Institute for Health and Care Excellence, aka 'NICE'. Not exactly cheap as chips, then...

***

I read a tweet which left me scratching my head bemusedly, on 9 October 2021. Written by someone styling himself 'Chris Wick News', @ChrisWickNews' :

It's almost been 3 years since I declined to be poisoned, cut or burned for my 'cancer'. I've now lived 2 years past the expiration date I was given.

The tweet had gathered 2,010 'likes', usually showing approval.

It rankled with me. On his introductory page, Mr Wick had amassed 19.6K 'followers' and described himself as 'An Independent Journalist and Truthseeker...SILANCE (sic) = DEATH.'

Where to start? Looking at his timeline I deduced that he is American.

I can barely begin to start to explain how I felt about his tweet.

I don't know which 'cancer' he was talking about but, if he is suggesting he doesn't believe there is any such thing as cancer - and otherwise why apostrophise it? – why is he boasting about living a couple of years beyond his 'expiration' date, because presumably there was nothing wrong with him in the first place?

If he is not prepared to accept there is anything which qualifies to be called cancer, why even go to see a doctor?

***

Tragically, on 15 October 2021, MP Sir David Amess was murdered. He was Patron of PC charity, Prost8, which declared:

'Every member of the Prost8 charity team are saddened and

distraught at the news of the tragic passing of our amazing and hardworking patron, Sir David Amess MP.

All thoughts and prayers are with Sir David's family, friends, colleagues and all who knew, loved and respected him.

Our work will continue in his name and we will strive even harder to make him proud of our achievements.'

As I finished off the book, and with final draft stage approaching, in mid November, former England cricketer, Alan Lamb, now 67, revealed he had PC: 'You don't usually want to put stuff on social media about your health,but I think it's so important. If I can save lives and get the awareness out to people, then I'm all for it.'

***

An update regarding the future – if it had one – of Mount V appeared in my local paper – well, what passed for that description these days. It, like so many now, was extremely unlike the way local papers used to be, particularly the one where I had begun my journalistic career in the late '60s.

In those days, and until relatively recently, local papers carried local news sourced by reporters, rather than just regurgitating press releases from the local council and advertisers, as appeared to be the norm now.

Anyway, I digress, as I so often do, but for once there was a genuine story. This one with a byline stating Adam Shaw as the author, who was described as a 'local democracy reporter'. 'Local', okay, I could just about accept that, even in a paper often featuring 'stories' not remotely to do with the town whose name the *Harrow Times* bears. 'Reporter' – no complaint about that, but 'democracy'... Democracy reporter... *What* was that supposed to mean?

However, the headline over the piece, datelined 6 August 2021, was this: 'Mount Vernon Cancer Centre needs £300m...'. And the subheading: 'Bids for government cash are an option'.

The story explained that Mount V was 'relying on £272 million to fund a transfer to Watford General Hospital', and added that it served a catchment area of 'almost 2 million people, with more than 5,000 new patients registered every year'. It added that 'NHS bosses' were intending 'to bid for government support under a new health plan that will aid eight new schemes across England'. Submissions would be accepted in September with a final decision on whether the application would be granted due in spring of 2022. Nothing I read changed my opinion that a refurbishment of Mount V where it was, and had been for so long, would actually be the best outcome for the most people and patients, though this had now been virtually written off as an option.

My MP David Simmonds wrote to me again a fortnight later:

The review of the cancer centre at Mount Vernon continues, and there is not a great deal to report at this stage. As I have said previously, the clinical need to relocate to a new site is a compelling argument and one which I can understand.

However, since I last wrote on this matter there have been a few issues which have cropped up and have made it clear that these changes are not going to be taking place at quite the pace people had previously worried.

The first is that the Paul Strickland Scanner Centre, which provides an essential service to the cancer centre, is an entirely separate charity with its own equipment and so cannot be easily included in the move.

The second element is that, while the clinical case for a move is strong, the project does not currently have any funding signed off. As such, once the review has concluded, a full business case will need to be presented to the Department for Health and Social Care before it can be progressed.

The positive side to all this is that it gives us the time to ensure this is all done correctly, and we can help alleviate the concerns that residents have raised previously. I am hoping to meet with the team again in the near future and I shall be working with them to ensure we deliver the best outcomes for patients.

I remain unconvinced that it would be in most patients' best interests to remove this incredible asset from the grounds where it has established itself and its amazing team of medics over so many years.

Of course, the fact that it is the place where I was treated with such professionalism, care and respect cannot help but colour my opinion of its merits. However, during the course of writing this book, I came across virtually no criticism of this admittedly far from immaculately housed institution, but one so full of heart and humour, not to mention hard-working staff. I observed them helping all patients selflessly, tirelessly and brilliantly, regardless of their age, attitude, sex, race or appearance.

Mount Vernon, I knew you intimately for only three months, but in that time, you experienced all of my mood swings with understanding, patience and positivity.

I prostrate myself before you and those who work within you.

THE END

ACKNOWLEDGEMENTS

*MANY thanks to all those who have helped me before, during and after the events described in these pages.

*FRIENDS and family who suffered my even more variable than usual mood swings. Unbelievably, none had a go at me – even those who didn't know why.

*EVERYONE who spoke to me about their experiences with and from the effects of PC.

*MY fellow patients, who must have had similar thoughts about me as I did about them, without being able to reveal them in a book.

*THE MEDICS, who treated me with nothing but respect, courtesy, expertise and overwhelmingly good humour – yes, except that one...

*SHEILA. GRAHAM BROWN. RON.

'A mesmerizing blend of memoir, travel, music and social history'
– *The Vinyl District*

'This amusing, entertaining and warm tome is a semi-autobiographical love letter to records, record collecting/collectors, and second-hand record shops' – *The Journalist*

'This book is a love letter to record collecting and the record shops that feed the addictions of those who have fallen under the spell of vinyl' – *Every Record Tells A Story*

'*Vinyl Countdown* has a lot of humour, good vibrations and a complete lack of self-importance and show off... Sharpe has a chatty, easy style'
– *NB Magazine*

'A wonderful mix of travelogue and musical knowledge'
– **Johnnie Walker,** *BBC Radio 2 – Sounds of the 70s*

'Hugely enjoyable' – *The Led Zeppelin Magazine*

'A nostalgic blend of memoir and social history that follows Graham's ongoing odyssey exploring the nation's record shops'
– *Choice Magazine*

'An engaging rummage around a lifetime's collecting... breathtakingly comprehensive' – *Record Collector Magazine*

'An entertaining read...' – *Shindig*

'Freighted with encyclopaedic knowledge, this intriguing tome encapsulates an unshakeable sense of purpose and often extraordinary encounters' – *Rock 'N' Reel*